BOOT CAMP abs

BOOT CAMP
abs

Get Rock-Hard Abs
with Former Marine Captain Charla McMillian

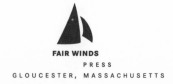

FAIR WINDS
PRESS
GLOUCESTER, MASSACHUSETTS

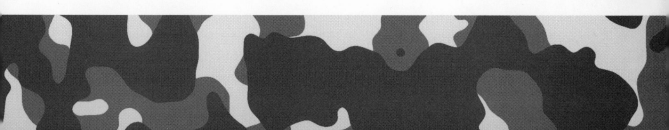

First published in the USA in 2005 by
Fair Winds Press
33 Commercial Street
Gloucester, MA 01930
09 08 07 06 05   1 2 3 4 5
ISBN 1-59233-125-4
Library of Congress Cataloging-in-Publication Data available

Cover and interior design by John Hall Design Group, www.johnhalldesign.com
Photography by Allan Penn Photography
Printed and bound in Canada

The information in this book is for educational purposes only. It is not intended to replace the
advice of a physician or medical practitioner. Please see your health care provider before
beginning any new health program.

To Mom. You taught me straightforward expression, strong leadership, effective teaching and coaching, commitment to excellence, and goal focus before the Marine Corps even got the chance. I know you can read this from Heaven. I hope you like it.

contents

acknowledgments

I am grateful to so many people for the opportunity to package my training concepts into this book and for its successful completion. I am also very thankful for the chance to help more people improve their lifestyle, physical performance, health and physique through this work.

Special thanks to Braden "Vegas" Plant for introducing me to the fine folks at Rockport Publishers where this all began. Thanks to Paul "4" Riley, my excellent co-model for all the photos, for being willing to show off what FitBoot training and all the advice in this book can really produce. Thank you to my outstanding editor Donna and her editorial staff for all the guidance and for ultimately pulling this whole thing together. Kudos to the photographers for capturing the hard work while helping to make the smiles genuine. And special thanks to my partner, "Fire" for the faith and encouragement, patience, and for helping to ensure that this book makes its way to everyone who needs it. Thank you all.

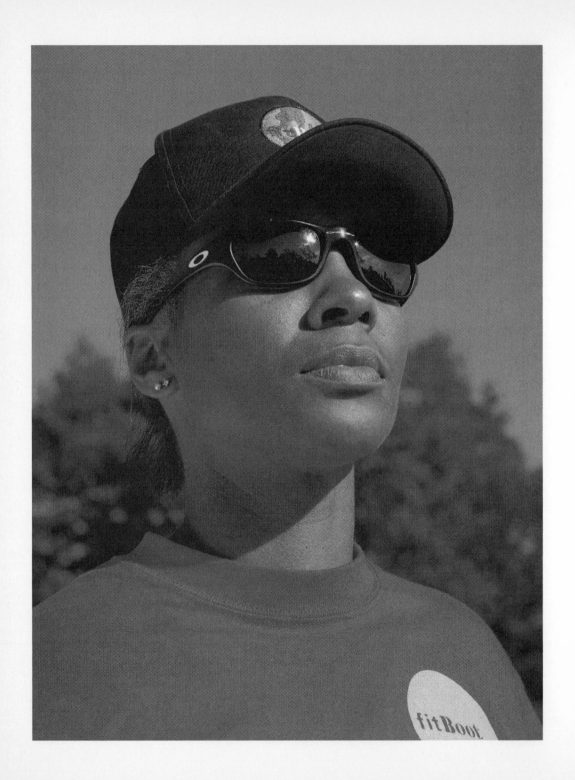

about the author

Since 1997, I have been teaching Boston-area executives, and housewives, competitive athletes, graduate students, couch potatoes and law enforcement and military candidates to eat better, train smarter, and realize their physique and performance potential. As a National Strength and Conditioning Association (NSCA)-certified specialist, I bring the credentials of one of only three accredited certifying organizations for fitness professionals to my work as a personal trainer and owner of FitBoot—Basic Training for Professionals, New England's original boot camp fitness program.

But the story began much earlier.

In high school, I competed on the boys' varsity cross-country team. Although I've never had any particular passion for distance running, my beloved South Carolina prep school was too small to field either a girls' track or cross-country team, so I ran on the boys' cross-country team. During that time, I also developed a love for improving my strength with resistance training in the gym and honed my power by doing interval sprints before and after cross-country practice.

Then I went to college, where I did not join a sports team but enjoyed new academic pursuits, an active social life, and the misguided belief that I could keep eating whatever I wanted, occasionally play some recreational games, yet retain my shape. And I put on the

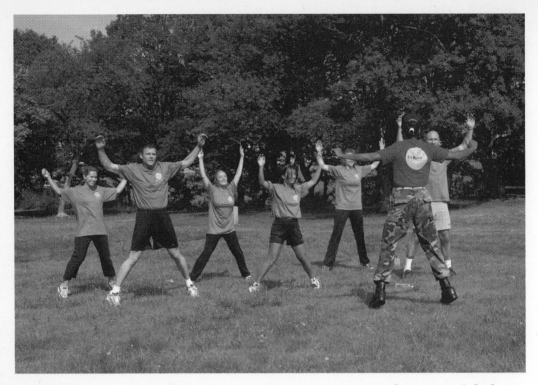

"Freshman 25"! Without structured team practice and my mom's balanced meals, I rapidly spiraled downward.

Finally, I got back in the gym. I began to read whatever I could get my hands on about fitness training. I hit the track as I had in high school. I stopped going back for seconds and thirds, late night pizza, and cider and doughnuts at Dartmouth's bountiful dining halls. And I regained my athletic physique.

Soon, my friends were seeking my advice on training routines and techniques. We all looked and felt a great deal better.

After graduating from college, I spent three fantastic months clarifying my thoughts, singing for my supper in the streets of Paris, and brainstorming career ideas. I came to the conclusion that I wanted to work in a field where both physical prowess and mental acuity were daily requirements. When I returned to the states, I called the local

U.S. Marine Corps recruiter and announced that I wanted to be an officer. Research at my college's career services center had shown me that the Corps offered my ideal balance: a job that demanded both brains and brawn, a legacy of the highest standards in both presentation and performance, and an established reputation as the best in the world at all that they do.

I was commissioned a second lieutenant on December 9, 1996. The next year, after completing training in Quantico, Virginia, I shipped out to my duty station at the Intelligence Analysis Unit for the First Marine Division, in Camp Pendleton, California, for the proudest two and a half years of my young life. I wore the uniform of the World's Finest. I dutifully studied and learned and briefed the division, base, and subordinate unit commanders on tactical threat levels, military capabilities, and likely responses to proposed military actions. I also supplemented my duties as military leader and mentor for my troops with time spent as their fitness trainer.

Every Marine unit's professional performance reflects the guidance and capabilities of its leaders. Military intelligence units often experience a reputation as having more brain but less brawn than their more field-ready counterparts. For a Marine, that's not a good thing. So I set out to ensure that Marines in the intelligence unit performed as well on the athletic field as they did in the briefing rooms.

I taught the men and women in my unit how to build flexibility, strength, and endurance along with good research, writing, and presentation skills. And I insisted on proper exercise technique along with proper rest, recovery, and good nutrition. I was proud of the results: consistently high fitness marks for my Marines and top physical fitness test honors for myself. I even scored perfectly on events then reserved for men, performing 80 sit-ups in two minutes and 20 pull-ups.

I left active duty in 1990 to get my Juris Doctor at Boston University School of Law. While I studied, I stayed physically active as the weekend supervisor at a local gym. All the while, I entertained the idea of starting a military-style exercise program for civilians. Over the next seven years, I constantly heard the same reaction from new friends and acquaintances as they learned of my service background: "Wow, the Marine Corps! I wish I could get in that kind of shape!" So in 1997, I created a way for civilians to get Marine-quality results— and FitBoot was born.

I earned my law degree because I found the study of law, like intelligence analysis, to be interesting and useful. I find my work as a fitness trainer, like the time I spent in a Marine Corps uniform, rewarding as a job that requires *mens sana in corpore sano,* a sound mind in a sound body.

I have earned my NSCA certification and have personally trained hundreds of civilians by balancing common military basic training drills and command voice discipline with professionally accepted strength and conditioning guidelines. And it works. So let's get you on the program!

introduction

So you want a flatter stomach, trimmer waist, and stronger core? Good idea. Your midsection holds the keys to a proud posture, a healthy pain-free back, and balanced physical performance at everything from playing with the kids to sprinting in out of the rain, from unloading the groceries to scoring the winning run at softball. It's also one of the toughest areas for most people to train—because you have to pay attention. Although you won't need to spend more than 15- to 20 minutes of each session focusing specifically on ab work, it's some of the most important training time you will log. You must learn how to properly isolate and flex your ab muscles and how to choose exercises that are appropriate for your current strength and endurance abilities. You also need to optimize your nutrition intake so that your efforts are visible. Consistency is a must. Most people don't have that kind of discipline. You're reading this, so you're telling me you're different.

Welcome to *Boot Camp Abs!*

IF YOU'RE READY TO STOP PLAYING with temporary solutions and half-stepping effort, you'll succeed with this program. If you're ready to get back to basics, get some work done, and get long-term results, then you should come along on this mission. But let's be very clear: If you're looking for total fitness in minutes or radical weight loss in days; if you're thinking of skimming over the instructions and doing *some* of what's required; if you're still focused on miracle results with minimal exertion and no discipline; then put this book down. Yes, you read that right. Put it down! Put it back on the shelf for someone who's ready to make real changes for consistent progress. Don't waste your time or money.

However, if you're ready to succeed, keep reading.

Regardless of the other training you do (and you need to keep up with your other training), you will now include targeted abdominal strength work on at least four days each week. It will take only 15- to 20 minutes of your daily training time, but it will provide an invaluable benefit for improving both your performance and appearance.

If your routine already includes substantial cardio work, but you've reached a plateau in body fat loss, endurance improvements, and/or speed, substitute only the aerobic training prescribed in this program for six to twelve weeks. You should then see significant improvements whether you return to your previous cardio routine or simply augment the plans found here.

Finally, in one place, you'll find how to train effectively without elaborate equipment, how to eat properly without crazy diets, and how to start balancing your optimized training and nutrition with adequate rest and recovery where all the improvements take place.

We'll begin by laying down some ground rules and debunking some popular myths around achieving all of your fitness goals.

First, keep it simple

On military briefing maps, playing fields, and battlefields, one rule stays constant: K.I.S.S. It stands for "Keep It Simple, Stupid!" No matter how difficult the goals may seem or how complex the mission, we succeed only by breaking large jobs into smaller, relatively simple tasks and then using common sense to complete them step by step. You have to understand what to do for specific goals and why those tasks make sense for you.

The principle has been the same for warriors since Napoleon's legendary battle plan tests. The story goes that, after hatching a new tactical scheme, Napoleon would summon a relatively inexperienced corporal in his army. Napoleon would describe the battle plan to this subordinate and then ask whether the man understood his instructions. If the corporal could follow the commander's intent, the plan would be implemented. If not, it was deemed too complex and doomed to failure, and Napoleon would simplify his strategy.

When we keep your training and other lifestyle improvements simple, you will be able to meet the requirements and remain consistent because you can understand the principles involved. This program involves simple principles, simple exercises, simple nutrition changes, and simple lifestyle improvements. It's the only smart game plan: common sense teamed with proven science, which you're encouraged to review for yourself. To guarantee your success, we have to keep it all simple.

But don't confuse simplicity with lack of detail. If we sacrifice accuracy and background information just to keep things simple, you're headed on a suicide mission. Napoleon couldn't strip his battle plan of critical details about the enemy, the area, or his planned movements and still expect to triumph in the war. Your situation is no different. You will succeed on your mission only if you understand the basics. To project confidence, feel energetic, look good, and perform well for the rest of your life, you'd better master the battle plan. We will follow the K.I.S.S. rule, without omitting anything of tactical significance.

Here's another simple concept: You need to work hard and stop looking for the quick, easy way out. The idea is so simple it evades most people.

Every day, you're bombarded with advice on how to make everything in your life easier. Television infomercials, radio spots, magazine ads, newspaper articles, coupons, and flyers all tout ways you can avoid any effort in your daily tasks.

FACT

A 1997 survey indicated that half of all American households contain at least one piece of exercise equipment. The same survey showed only about 2/3 of those pieces of equipment actually being used for exercise in the home.

SOURCE: Survey by Fitness Products Council, North Palm Beach, Florida

Despite most people's negative experience with fad diets, Americans keep buying the hype. According to a March 1999 report from CNN, of the 82% of consumers who agree that the USDA Food Pyramid (which advocates a carbohydrate based diet,) is the basis for healthy eating, 40% have tried a high-protein, low-carb diet. Of those, 40% gained some, all, or more of the weight back when they had to come off the diet while only 15% of those who lost weight following the USDA recommendations gained it back.

Use your common sense. Finding the easy way out has never been the strategy of anyone who does anything worthwhile.

These shortcuts work. Extremely restricted calories, madcap workouts, the latest gadget...it all works. But nothing works for long. You can do almost anything different from what you're doing now and you will see some quick results. But fads and quick fixes won't get you results you can keep. And if you've done something silly enough, you'll likely hurt yourself and have to stop training altogether, delaying your journey to real success.

orientation

So are you ready to reject the waste and failure of fads, magical results, and easy fixes? How about using some common sense and good judgment? Add in some discipline and mission-focus and you're on your way. Sound simple? You just might be catching on. Count yourself in on the road to fitness success—you're a Recruit completing *Boot Camp Abs*.

Report for Duty, Recruit!

YOUR QUEST FOR TOTAL FITNESS, lifestyle improvement, and attitude adjustment is just like any other tactical mission: It requires preparation, information, step-by-step planning, personal accountability, and the drive to attain the goal. Every mission begins with an order, and this book will provide you with yours.

In addition, you have your Recruit Field Journal, which will serve as your training journal, nutrition log, progress gauge, and quick reference manual. Have your Recruit Field Journal accessible at all times to record your requirements and review your success.

On your way, be sure you understand the information provided in each section of this book. If not, read it again and again until you do. Keep yourself honest by checking off each day's training session when you complete it . You wouldn't conduct any of your other business without monitoring projections, expectations, status, and progress. You won't neglect those details on this mission either. Once you spend a little time mapping out your plan and understanding the instructions, it shouldn't take long to record your daily nutrition and scheduled progress checks. Successfully completing your mission will justify your efforts. Use your brain, take action, and track your improvements!

One fundamental feature of FitBoot training that isn't always a part of other fitness programs I've seen, including "boot camps," is that I expect recruits to learn how to perform the drills, but also understand why we train the way we do. You should never accept "because I told you to" as any instructor's response to your serious questions or "because you're weak" as an explanation for alarming pain or lack of progress. Answers like that usually indicate that the instructor is what Marine intelligence analysts call a "hip-shooter," someone who'll make up the analysis he doesn't know—a real danger to the troops who rely on that information. Every training drill, diet change, and habit adjustment you're advised to make must have an identifiable purpose and reliable science behind it that you can comprehend.

Now, I can't stress enough the requirement for discipline. When I tell a FitBoot squad to jump, no one wastes my time asking "how high?" But they also learn why we jump, where jumping skill and power might be applicable, and how jumping fits into the rest of their training. Think about how your training helps you perform your daily activities better and how your improvements boost your self-confidence and energy levels. Consider how your improved nutrition contributes to your physical and mental prowess. When your thinking leads to other questions, then you need to explore the additional resources provided in the Reference section to get answers.

Ab Training Q&A

LET'S START WITH SOME BASIC QUESTIONS we need to answer and some common myths about abdominal training and development that we need to debunk.

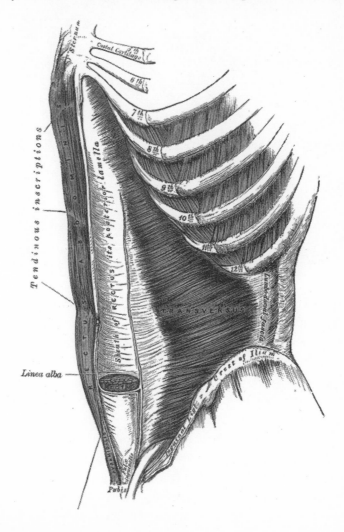

1) What are the abs? And why do some people get a six-pack?

Your midsection has two large muscle groups which make up what we typically

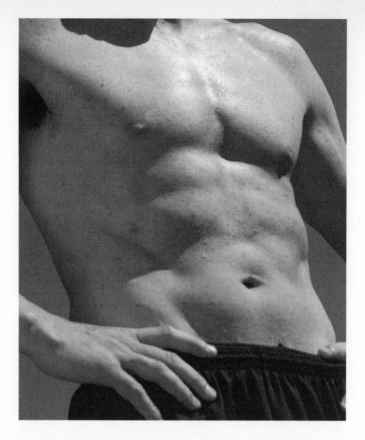

call the abdominals or abs, for short: the rectus abdominis (what most of us visualize when we think of abs) and the external obliques (often obscured by those annoying love handles). Developing a third muscle, the serratus anterior, which is actually part of the chest, can help fill out the picture on a truly well-defined torso if visual appeal is one of your goals.

Many athletes spend all their training time doing a few simple exercises for the rectus abdominis, the large muscle along the front of your midsection. The rectus abdominis is divided by several fibrous bands that run horizontally across the front of the ab wall. Typically, three of these "tendinous inscriptions" visibly divide the ab wall into rows, but some folks have one or two more bands that may be visible below the navel. In addition, another large tendon runs vertically down the middle of the wall, dividing it in half. The rectus abdominis and its tendon fibers show off the "six-pack" on a lean, well-trained physique. Although it is possible, in any given exercise, to engage more or fewer of the many fibers that make up this long flat muscle, it is still just one muscle.

Folks are also impressed when they can see your external obliques. The fibers of these muscles run along the sides of your torso, diagonally downward from near the bottom of your rib cage to the top of your hip bones (the iliac crest). An athlete with sufficiently low body fat may be able to display the indentations of these muscle fibers which appear like small diagonal "fingers" along the sides of the midsection.

The transversus abdominis is the most deeply buried of the ab muscles and is, therefore, not visible at the surface. You will not perform separate exercises or work to build any measurable size or definition for this muscle, but you must focus on engaging it at the start of every exercise because its split second contraction precedes full and proper flexing of the other ab muscles. Running beneath the rectus abdominis all the way down to the iliac crest, the transversus helps stabilize your back and pelvis all day long while you stand, sit, and walk and keeps you standing strong and unscathed if you play sports.

The serratus anterior is actually part of the chest region of muscles; however, because it starts from about your second or third rib at each side of your chest and runs diagonally downward and into the external obliques, keeping it strong and well-defined can really help improve that ab picture. Because we focus only on abs during this mission, your orders will not include chest exercises. But you need to include work for the chest along with all other major muscle groups in your overall training plans.

2) What do the abs do?

By now, most people know that they need strong abs for proper back support and good posture. That's great, but what does that mean exactly in terms of your ab training?

The job of every major muscle is to move a part of your body. The abs curve your spine. The rectus abdominis (remember the flat muscle along the front of your torso?) curves your spine forward, bringing your upper torso closer to your pelvis. The external obliques work to bend your spine slightly to the side. Those muscles flex to bend your torso over with a slight twist toward the front of your body. The transversus abdominis, properly focused on as you suck in that gut at the start of each exercise repetition, stabilizes your pelvis and spine and allows you to fully flex the more prominent ab muscles.

3) What are the most important things I can do for my abs?

First things, first, Recruit. Learn to stand up straight. You can start working your abs by gently engaging them all day long. As you walk around, sit at your desk or pick up one of the kids, focus often on keeping your chest and rib cage slightly expanded (the ab wall automatically flattens out a bit), shoulders relaxed and pulled back, and lower ab wall tight toward your spine. By doing so, you will continually use these muscles and help save your spine and the ligaments in your back from having to absorb body weight and lifting impact that they're not designed to handle.

Once you start training your abs properly, you will invoke that same good posture so that you can isolate them as much as possible while performing each exercise. You will learn to flex your abs as hard as you can without straining your back or pulling excessively with your legs (hip flexors) which would just defeat your purpose, waste your time, and likely get you hurt.

4) Do you need to do hundreds of sit-ups and crunches every day to have strong, good-looking abs?

No. All the muscles in your body respond similarly to training stimulus—the abs are no different. Very few people think they need to do hundreds of bench presses daily to get a strong chest or run hundreds of miles to get a strong heart and leg muscles. When you properly complete well chosen exercises, using good form and full range of motion for an appropriate number of repetitions, the muscles involved will get stronger and can increase in size. When you implement an appropriate nutrition plan, you will reduce that body fat to display your hard work as well.

Frankly, the vast majority of people I run across who claim to execute hundreds of sit-ups, crunches, leg raises, etc., every day are just wasting their time with momentum and movements involving every muscle *but* their abs. I usually challenge them to execute a few sets of ten repetitions after I teach them proper form and watch their incentive to count higher than 100 disappear.

5) Shouldn't I use weights to train the abs just as I do the other muscles?

For most people, probably not. Now pay attention, because this answer has an exception. Most recreational athletes are looking for a trimmer waist and a strong, flat ab wall. Progressive resistance work with weights usually induces some level of muscle growth (hypertrophy); the muscle fibers grow in size. For many people, causing too much hypertrophy in the abs equates to a thickening at the waist. Of course, your abs will be strong, but you probably do not want to see that area increase in size. Sticking with the weight of your own torso as you work to flex these muscles should provide sufficient resistance for growth and strength improvements without widening your waistline.

What's the exception? Athletes who play contact sports, especially those involving potential hits from the side and rapid changes of direction. For these athletes, performance is usually more important than a specific look. If you play football, rugby, Aussie rules football, wrestling, or ice hockey, your sport often involves the need to physically resist the body weight of another person with your torso or to move another player using force generated at your midsection. You will be better protected by abdominal muscles strengthened using some resistance work (i.e.: weights, other people, rubber bands) to help prevent unexpected jolts to your back and potentially injurious twists and bends at the spine.

6) Don't I need that special rolling-swinging-rocking thing I saw advertised on TV to get the most out of my ab training?

No. Here's the beauty of boot camp training. You will quickly learn that you need nothing more than your own body weight and solid ground beneath you to make significant improvements in your performance and physique. Add a bench or chair and possibly a chin-up bar and you multiply your possibilities. But recent tests done using the most famous commercially advertised portable ab training devices showed that only one helped the user engage the abdominal muscles more than traditional crunches. And the one that did add more work did so by adding resistance to the crunch motion, a practice that may not be suitable for all athletes for the reasons discussed in the answer to the previous question.

Don't get me wrong: Progressive resistance training with free weights, machines, elastic bands, or growing children is extremely valuable for improving strength and sculpting muscle. It's just not the only answer. And this is especially true for abs, where excess hypertrophy is not usually a goal, it's not always desirable. Simply learning to properly flex your ab muscles and use their full range of motion for each exercise will help you achieve your goals.

7) If I've got love handles and a flabby gut, don't I just need to do more sit-ups to get good abs?

Well, yes and no. Keep in mind that you have two missions here: First, to strengthen and develop your ab wall so that it looks and performs well for the sports and activities you do; and second, to reduce your body fat so that you can see the results of your efforts. There are many athletes whose conditioning work has given them strong midsections. And if you touch the muscles in their torsos, you can feel that they are hard and strong, maybe even well-defined by the tendons that run laterally and along the midline. But you can't see the definition because there's still too much flab surrounding the area.

That's where nutrition comes into play. Increasing the number of reps you do will not reduce the love handles and the general softness of the surrounding area. The amount of body fat has to come down. But there's no such thing as "spot-reducing" (being able to choose the area from which the body burns the fat you need to lose). You didn't get to choose where the flab went, and you don't get to determine

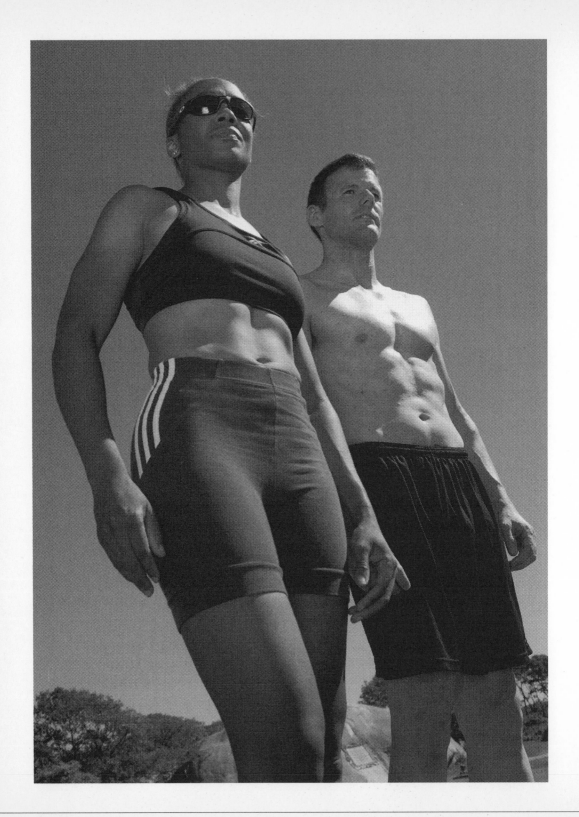

where or in what order it will burn off. But by working to optimize your whole body nutrition and ensuring that you perform the appropriate aerobic exercise, you will help speed your metabolism, burn off excess fat, and improve your odds of seeing those sculpted abs.

8) I'm a guy and I want my abs "jacked," but my girlfriend just needs to tone and flatten her abs. Don't we need completely different training routines?

The short answer? No. That distinction is just the stuff of magazine covers luring you to buy another issue every month. Unless your girlfriend has an abnormally high level of testosterone or you have atypically high estrogen levels, the natural genetic differences between men and women will dictate the slightly different ways in which you will develop with the same training.

The higher levels of the hormone estrogen in women give them more body fat and less muscle mass than men. Consistent, targeted abdominal strength training will help both men and women develop some muscularity in that area; as with every muscle, males have the potential to build larger fibers than their female counterparts. Optimized nutrition and good aerobic training will help women lower their body fat percentage to help make those ab muscles more visible, but they will generally still carry more body fat above the waist than the men. Males will typically carry less body fat and will, therefore, likely display more definition of those well-trained abs (to look "jacked").

Keep in mind that there is actually no training result scientifically known as "toning." The only possible outcomes from your work are increases in muscular strength, increases in muscle fiber size (hypertrophy), and/or increases in muscular endurance. Although muscle tone is certainly improved with good strength and conditioning work, "toning" is just a term coined by fitness industry salesmen to counter many females' fear of going to the gym because they might become too muscular. Consider your true goals: muscular hypertrophy (*slightly* increasing the size of your abdominal muscles) and aerobic exercise to help you lose enough body fat to see those results.

Questions answered? Good.
Stand by to execute...turn the page, and begin!

Report to Medical

BEFORE ANY UNIT SHIPS OUT, the commander inspects the troops, assessing their physical and mental readiness to execute the mission. Whether reporting for military training or starting an exercise program, you have to make sure you can handle the training. Even if you think you're in good health, you may have forgotten prior injuries, illnesses, or family health history that warrant caution or modification of your activities. As much as I'd like to bring every available body along on this mission, you won't keep up or achieve your objective if you get hurt because you skipped your med check.

For starters, review your personal risk factors. These risks and history may send up a red flag that you need medical clearance and/or supervision when training. Check off all of the following that apply to you.

- ❐ **Are you older than 40?**

- ❐ **Do you have any history of cardiovascular disease?**

- ❐ **Has your doctor ever indicated that you have heart trouble or a heart murmur?**

- ❐ **Have you had a heart attack?**

- ❐ **Do you get any chest pains while resting or when exerting yourself *or* do you frequently feel pains or pressure in the left (or midchest) area, left neck, shoulder, or arm during or immediately following exertion?**

- ❐ **Has anyone in your family developed coronary heart disease before the age of 55 *or* did your father, mother, brother, or sister have a heart attack before age 50?**

- ❐ **Is your total cholesterol level higher than 200?**

- ❐ **Have you ever had an abnormal electrocardiogram (ECG/EKG) or any history of abnormal heart rhythms?**

- ❐ **Do you experience extreme breathlessness after mild exertion?**

- ❐ **Do you smoke?**

- ❐ **Have you ever been told you have high blood pressure or dangerously low blood pressure *or* do you not know whether your blood pressure is normal?**

☐ Have you ever had any joint problems or any injury to your bones or joints, including arthritis, chondromalacia, or osteoporosis?

☐ Do you have any chronic muscular problems?

☐ Are you currently pregnant or have you delivered within the past three months?

☐ Have you recently had surgery?

☐ Do you have a history of diabetes or hypoglycemia?

☐ Do you have asthma?

☐ Have you been physically inactive for more than six months?

☐ Are you more than 20 pounds over your ideal weight? (See height/weight chart in the Recruit Field Journal, page 155.)

☐ Do you have a medical condition not mentioned here that might need special attention in an exercise program? (For example, chronic fatigue syndrome, fibromylagia, physical disability, kidney or other internal organ problems.)

If you answer in the affirmative for any of these listed risk factors, you must check in at sick bay before you begin training. Sounds like a pain in the rear end, right? Or, maybe you figure you can bypass the med check because you feel fine and nothing has happened the other hundred times you've tried to get in shape? This time around, act with good sense! Every hard-body you've admired running in perfect step in a platoon formation or standing fit and strong in dress blues had to clear a medical check before they could even get on the bus. You're not uniquely qualified and you won't get special treatment here, Recruit. Go see the doc!

Once you have the thumbs up to begin, you have to mark your starting point. You will now evaluate your current fitness level, in this case measuring abdominal strength and endurance only, for a reality check of your strength and coordination and a baseline for gauging your progress. Remember, this is where you're *starting*. If you score well, you can immediately set your sights on excellence. If not, you'll be highly motivated to get your work done and keep reaching higher. And you should be proud every time you see any improvement.

Fitness Assessment

ALL RIGHT, RECRUIT, get ready to take a portion of the same test we use to evaluate FitBoot recruits. Be advised: No basic fitness test can tell you everything about your health, physical fitness, or ability to play a sport or mow the grass. You'll measure your current body composition (fat and muscle) and your readiness to perform particular abdominal strength and endurance exercises. Every score—no matter how good or how poor—can be improved with focused training.

After recording your body composition information and performance level, you will determine the category of exercises appropriate for your ability. We'll borrow the skill designations used on Marine Corps shooting ranges: Marksman = Beginner; Sharpshooter = Moderate; Expert = Very Fit. You will execute the training plan that matches your skill designation and increase your challenges when you improve.

There is detail involved here, and you will need to exert yourself moderately to complete your assessment. You said you were ready to stop half-stepping, so let's get started, Recruit!

Break out your Recruit Field Journal and record your assessment information on the Initial Fitness Assessment Chart [page 149].

Vital Signs

On the Fitness Assessment Chart, list your age, height in inches, and weight in pounds. Remember that the best time to weigh yourself is first thing in the morning, just after you get up and make a head call (bathroom visit, Recruit) and before you get dressed or eat or drink anything. If you must choose a different time of day to weigh in, be sure to do future updates at the same time of day and in the same state of dress for consistency.

Record your most recent blood pressure reading on the Fitness Assessment chart. If you haven't had your blood pressure checked within the last year, get it checked now even if it was normal before.

Get your resting heart rate by taking your pulse. You will be most rested if you take it first thing in the morning before you get out of bed, but you can take it now if you are sitting comfortably and no one is screaming at you. You should take your pulse in one of two places: at your carotid artery by placing two fingers at the heel of your jawbone and pressing in lightly, or at your radial artery by placing two fingers on the inside of your wrist on the thumb side just inside your wrist bone. Don't use your thumb to take your pulse! The thumb has its own pulse, and your count will be wrong. Count for 30 seconds and multiply by two. Record your resting heart rate on your Fitness Assessment Chart.

Body Composition

Okay, Recruit, time to find out just how hard or soft you are. You will now choose a method to estimate how much body fat you're carrying. Keep yourself calm! First, remember some key information about body fat. You can't have 0%, so that's not a goal. Some body fat is essential. A small percentage is carried in the basic structure of your cells and around your internal organs to cushion and protect them from injury. The average female carries about 12 to 15% essential fat, while males carry about 3 to 5%. The rest is called "storage fat". You need some storage fat for energy reserves during intense physical activity and, for females, to maintain normal menstrual cycles. But, chances are, you probably don't need as much storage fat as you may be carrying. Regardless of the other objectives you identify, you will work to maintain optimal fat levels to improve your physical performance and enhance your physical appearance.

The only perfect way to determine how much of your body weight is fat would involve dissecting your body. Presumably, you don't want to do that, so the best you can do is estimate. Now this part involves detail, so put your thinking cap on. There are several different ways to evaluate your body composition, and each one uses different measurements, assumptions, and calculations. Some tests are more readily accessible than others, some have smaller margins of error and are therefore more reliable than others. The most commonly used methods, from most to least reliable, are:

> **hydrodensitometry or underwater weighing**

> **skinfold caliper testing**

> **bioelectrical impedance analysis**

> **tape measure circumference testing**

> **near infrared testing**

> **Body Mass Index (BMI) calculation**

> **waist-to-hip ratio calculation**

We will focus on the three most readily available methods from which you might choose.

Bioelectrical Impedance Analysis

In bioelectrical impedance analysis or BIA, a low voltage electrical current is sent through your body via electrodes touching the skin. (Heads up! If you wear a pacemaker or other internal electrical device, you *cannot* use this method.) As you remember from grade school science class, salt water, which is the water found in your body, conducts electricity. Muscle contains more water than fat (70% versus 5 to 13%), so the leaner you are, the faster the electrical current travels. The whole process takes only a few seconds. Your age, height, total body weight, and gender all factor into the average amount of water your body should contain. The tester feeds that data into the BIA device which calculates your body fat percentage. As long as you are normally hydrated and have controlled all variables, BIA is very reliable except with the extremely obese and the extremely lean.

BOTTOM LINE: BIA testing measures how quickly your body conducts an electrical current to estimate lean body mass. The speed, portability, and non-invasive nature of the test make it more accessible than many other methods.

PROBLEMS: The test is only reliable if your body has a normal amount of water in it. The equations used in these tests can overestimate the amount of fat in a very lean body and underestimate the fat in an obese body. A recent study also found that BIA seriously underestimates body fat in women who carry excess weight in the lower body. Consuming alcohol, caffeine, or other diuretics within 24 hours before testing can dehydrate you and skew the test results. BIA can also be affected by your body position, the presence of metallic jewelry, your body temperature, the use of oral contraceptives, and recent exercise. It's a convenient test, but it can be easily confused.

MARGIN OF ERROR: +/- 3 to 5%

FACT

You don't need to find a lab to have your body fat estimated with BIA, but you may need to shop around. I use a small hand-held BIA device to estimate body fat percentages in myself and my clients. Available for about $150 at such stores as The Sharper Image and Brookstone, this device works well for estimating and monitoring relative changes in most people. I have not been as pleased with the results from BIA scales you can buy for home use. I don't know of any controlled studies of the home scales, but my clients who own them often report body fat percentages that don't match the individuals' physical appearance.

FACT

I've had clients who were tested at big-name health clubs using commercial versions of BIA devices. Some of these clubs seem to make a policy of telling all new members they're ridiculously fat! I wasn't present, so I don't know whether the testers were inexperienced, whether the clients were improperly hydrated, whether electrodes were properly placed, etc., but I do know that a 5'4" female who weighs 125 pounds, follows a sensible nutrition plan, plays competitive sports, and has a generally athletic appearance should not register 40% body fat unless something is terribly wrong with the test. If you choose BIA and get illogical results, buy a better quality device or find a facility that is more interested in science and accuracy than membership fees.

Body Mass Index

Your height and weight are used to develop a ratio that tells whether you're obese. This ratio is called your Body Mass Index (BMI). These new guidelines, supported by the National Institutes for Health (NIH) and the National Heart, Lung, and Blood Institute (NHLBI), are used to identify individuals potentially at risk for obesity-related health problems and premature death. This method of estimating body composition was chosen because it is more comparable to the standards used by the rest of the Western world to identify obesity among the populations of nations. While BMI does not actually estimate your body fat percentage, it provides a guideline. If you are unable to get a body fat measurement, calculate your BMI as follows:

(Weight in pounds) ÷ (height in inches x height in inches) x 703

EXAMPLE: A female who is 5'4" (64") tall and weighs 130 pounds has a BMI of 22, as figured below:

64" x 64" = 4096

130 lbs. / 4096 = .031

.031 x 703 = 22 BMI

Go to the National Heart, Lungs, and Blood Institute Web site (http://www.nhlbi.nih.gov/guidelines/obesity/bmi_tbl.htm) to find a simple chart with BMI readings.

BOTTOM LINE: BMI is quick and easy to calculate.

PROBLEMS: Because BMI does not account for muscularity, it's not very helpful for athletes or for recording more than the most obvious physique improvements. If you're very muscular for your height, your BMI may indicate that you're obese even when you're clearly not. In addition, BMI is not accurate for those who are very short (i.e., under 5'0") or for the elderly who may lose muscle mass as they age.

Waist-to-Hip Ratio

The waist-to-hip ratio test indicates where body fat is primarily located and may be a good predictor of potential health risks. Some studies suggest that body shape can indicate where and what kind of excess fat the person carries. An apple-shaped body is wider in the middle than at the top and bottom. "Apples" seem to carry more fat around their internal organs (visceral fat) and could be at higher risk for diabetes, cardiovascular disease, and some cancers. A pear shape, in which the lower body is wider than the upper body appears to indicate lower health risks.

Knowing what fruit you resemble isn't really useful for recording specific body-fat changes, but it may be helpful for monitoring general physique improvements. Use the following method to find out where you fit in the produce department.

1) **Using a tape measure, measure your hips, in inches, at the widest point.**

2) **Measure your waist, in inches, at the narrowest point (usually about halfway between your navel and the bottom of your sternum, that narrow bone at the center of your chest. You may have to try a few spots above your hip bone to get the lowest number).**

3) **Divide the number from Step 2 by the number from Step 1. The result is your weight to height ratio.**

BOTTOM LINE: Waist-to-hip ratio is another fast, simple method for making basic predictions about your body composition. It may be helpful for noting general changes in your physical size.

PROBLEMS: This method will not tell you what percentage of your body is fat and may be even less reliable for determining the distribution of body fat in obese individuals. If you're attempting to obtain your measurements by yourself (i.e., without someone assisting), you're likely to get inaccurate numbers.

Choose a method and get your measurements right. Record your body composition information in your Recruit Field Journal and then move on to assess your physical ability.

Abdominal Strength and Endurance

During *Boot Camp Abs*, we will focus on what you can do to slim your waist and strengthen your midsection. Hopefully, you know by now that your quest for complete fitness must involve a balanced approach to both training and nutrition for the whole body. So while we keep the abs under the microscope for this mission, you'd better be thinking about a good plan for strengthening every other muscle in your body as well, Recruit! For now, we'll evaluate your ab strength and endurance to find your initial ability level for training.

EXERCISE

Ground-Zero Estimate

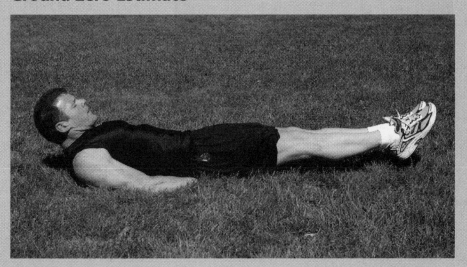

PREPARATION: If you have a buddy, have him or her use a ruler or tape measure to determine your ground-zero point. Without a buddy, you will estimate your ground zero by eyeballing how high your legs are off the ground.

Lie flat on your back with your arms flat down by your sides, legs raised straight up and perpendicular to the deck. In this position, your back should be completely flat with no arch or space between your lower back and the ground.

PROPER EXERCISE TECHNIQUE: Keeping your back flat, slowly lower your legs, keeping them straight and together, to the lowest point where your lower back remains perfectly flat with no arch at all. Hold that position for a few seconds to ensure that only your abs are flexed and that you can keep from arching your back.

DATA: If you have a buddy, have her measure the distance between your legs and the ground. If you are alone, raise your head slightly and estimate how many inches they are off the deck. Record your approximate or measured result in your Recruit Field Journal.

Timed Curl-ups:

PREPARATION: You'll need a stopwatch, a clock with a second hand, or an egg timer that you'll set for 60 seconds. If you have a buddy to help you, he or she can anchor your feet and mark the time. If you're training alone, locate a solid object that can anchor your feet (a sofa, weight bench, or door will do fine).

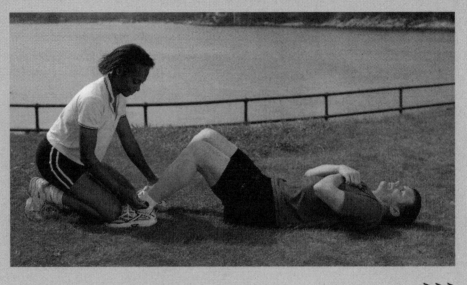

> > >

Presumably, you've survived your Fitness Assessment. Congratulations!

Now refer to the Fitness Test Scoring Charts in your Recruit Field Journal (page 147). The charts will help you determine whether you need to drop or gain some weight, lose some fat, or just keep getting stronger while maintaining your good physique. Locate and circle the skill designation that matches your abdominal strength and endurance test scores.

Now that you have a picture of your baseline, let me remind you again:

These scores and measurements mark your start point!

From here, you'll mark your progress toward your checkpoints and your objectives. Don't get your shorts in a knot over how bad (or how good) your initial scores are.

PROPER EXERCISE TECHNIQUE: Lie on your back on the deck with your feet flat and held down (by your buddy or the furniture), and knees bent. Cross your arms over your chest with hands on opposite shoulders and elbows in contact with your chest or rib cage. You will curl your torso and sit up, with no gap between your forearms and your rib cage, until your elbows touch your thighs, then uncurl so that your shoulder blades touch the deck. Do as many curl-ups as possible in one minute without bouncing off the deck, raising your hips to propel yourself up, or moving your arms. Stop after 1 minute.

DATA: Record the number of curl-ups you performed correctly within the time limit.

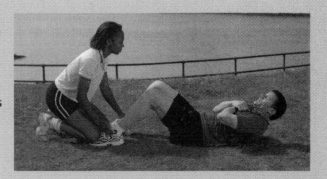

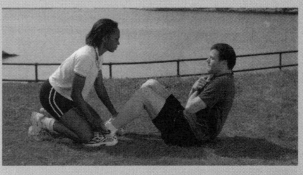

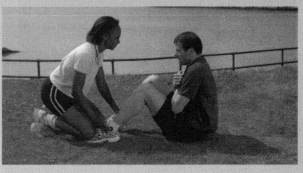

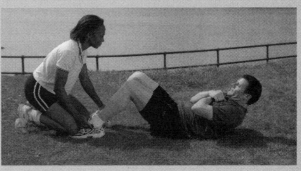

mission start

You know where you are. You've established where you need to go. Now, how do you get there?

It's time to execute the mission you've planned. You'll work to train a strong midsection using basic training exercises appropriate for your ability level. You will learn the fundamentals of nutrition, metabolism, and muscular development through training. You will work to improve your habits. In the process, you will strengthen your mind.

The Concept

TO REACH THE OBJECTIVES of this mission, you will complete ab strength training (including lower back work for balance) on 4 days a week and aerobic training 3 days each week. You must also rest at least 1 to 2 days each week. To continually improve your whole body, you will need to add work for your other major muscle groups 3 to 4 days a week, skills training (balance, agility, coordination, and any necessary sports techniques) at least once a week, and flexibility work at least 3 days a week.

Some folks might question whether they really need to include all these other training activities. They say, "What happened to just parking farther from the mall?"

Some solid answers come from the National Weight Control Registry (NWCR), a database maintained by Lifespan, part of Rhode Island's first Health System. This registry contains information on more than 4,000 adults who have lost at least 30 pounds and kept if off for at least one year. With periodic questionnaires and surveys, Lifespan's researchers have found that their average registrants have actually lost about 60 pounds each and kept if off for roughly five years. These successful people typically report burning an average of 2,800 calories per week by walking, climbing stairs, and increasing other activities along with participating in a variety of structured physical activities, including aerobic exercise and weight lifting. They typically stuck to a smart long-term diet, one that includes low-fat, lean protein, and high amounts of whole grains, fruits, and vegetables. (Fewer than 50% followed commercial diet programs.) This activity requirement is also now confirmed by the U.S. government's latest *Dietary Guidelines for Americans* 2005. In these recommendations the government now agrees that everyone needs to engage in 60 to 90 minutes of exercise daily and keep nutrition optimised like you will learn to do here to stay healthy and fit. In the end, real, structured, vigorous activity along with sensible attention to nutrition still wins as the key to success.

To get real results, you have to do real work. But do the math, Recruit! Unless you have 9 days in your weeks, then you'll have to combine activities on some days. If you can only dedicate 30 minutes a day, then you'll need to find that half hour on at least 5 days each week and divide your training plans into shorter segments to get all your work done. If you have committed to 45 to 60 minute training sessions, then you can train a minimum of 3 days weekly (although an additional day or two won't kill you). Renew your commitment to well-rounded conditioning; you can achieve the minimal benefits with fewer training days and less time and effort, but you'll need an extra push to achieve your potential.

Here's the intel on what you get from this basic training. You need strength training to improve your ability to move your own body weight and other objects. The muscular development you get from strength training helps you to shape your body, so it's not smaller but still flabby. Muscle gives your body contours, but fat just sits there. So if you don't see any definition after all your strength work, you've still got some fat to peel away. Strength training also raises your metabolic rate for up to 18 hours after you finish training, so your body's furnace keeps working to burn that excess fat even while you're resting.

Your strength improves when you consistently stimulate your muscles to perform more than they're used to doing—a principle known as "overload." To meet overload, you can challenge your muscles to move a gradually increasing resistance more often, or, in the case of the ab work you'll do here, to move at different angles more often for increased difficulty.

You need aerobic training to improve your cardiovascular endurance, which is achieved by overloading your heart and lungs and causing them to work harder than they would at rest. Improving your cardiovascular endurance will enable you to keep going—at whatever you're doing—longer. The American College of Sports Medicine (ACSM), the largest and one of the most respected sports medicine and exercise science organizations in the world, defines aerobic activity as "any activity that uses large muscle groups, can be maintained continuously, and is rhythmic in nature." The term "rhythmic" includes any ongoing, repetitive motion (like walking or running), so those of you who are "dance challenged" can still get your cardio work done! To fire up that metabolic furnace, you need aerobic exercise for 20 minutes to 1 hour, continuously, on 3 to 5 days each week. For our purposes, aerobic work is vital for helping to burn the fat that hides your muscular development. Your mission will include moderate intensity aerobic work on 2 training days with more intense effort on one day each week.

You will include flexibility training to preserve and improve the range of motion in your joints and muscles, help you avoid injury while training, and help you prepare your muscles for more vigorous activity. To improve your flexibility, you will choose two or three of your favorite stretches plus one or two that you usually hate (since that's probably an area you really need work on) and hold each stretch for 30 seconds at the end of every training session.

You will conduct your training "by the numbers." Beginning with exercises and repetitions that you can handle, you'll learn to push yourself just beyond your mental and physical comfort zone every training day. You'll learn to appreciate the difference between the mild, temporary discomfort of real effort and the danger-indicating pain of over exertion, and you will avoid the latter. Both your body and mind will learn to adapt and improve. When you can properly complete the top range of sets and reps within your skill designation without failure and without excessive soreness the next day, you will move to the next level. You will increase how much you do (training volume) and how hard you work at it (training intensity) using both the planned schedule and your common sense to gauge your improving abilities. You will NOT drag your feet!

But hold on a minute, Recruit. You will not rush off half-cocked to quickly increase your training intensity or volume, either. Your muscles—including your heart—will get stronger and begin to take shape in a relatively short time. The joints, ligaments, and tendons that hold the machine together don't get conditioned as quickly. You might make impressive strength gains in three or four weeks, but you'll set yourself up for injury if you don't give the connective tissues time to catch up. You will follow your training plans in the order listed to avoid injury.

By planning both training and recovery, you will advance step-by-step toward your objective. You'll make steady, predictable progress and steer clear of injuries and overtraining.

Every week during the six-week program, you will also review one of the Briefings in the Knowledge Chapter (page 83). Through these Briefings, you will bolster your understanding of basic concepts like nutrition and metabolism. Now, eager recruits will try to absorb all of the intel in one sitting. It won't work. You must take the time to understand the details and to gradually incorporate the required changes into your daily life. The Briefings are intended to help you negotiate the headlines, sound bites, and advertising hype that have confused you to this point. Treat them as classroom lessons and homework that, completed step-by-step, enable you to master a complicated topic by the end of the school term. On the first day of school, you wouldn't try to cover the whole reading list or take the final exam, so don't try to cover all your briefing information in one day or make drastic changes to your normal habits overnight.

The Tasks

ON THIS MISSION, you will use the FitBoot training that has helped people in the Boston area build great physiques. You will do some of the same exercises and drills used by Marines and other service members to get and stay in shape, plus additional strength-builders that I have developed and learned over the past few decades.

Your specific training plans are located in your Recruit Field Journal so that you can bring them with you to your training site and so that you can track important data about your nutrition habits and training progress. Your training plans list the exercises and drills you will execute each week.

Before you start your first full training session, take the time now to familiarize yourself with the exercises for your skill level and below—Marksman, Sharpshooter, or Expert. Then refer to the appropriate pages in your Recruit Field Journal (page 147) and familiarize yourself with the format of your training plans. When that's done, come back and finish reading the rest of your orders: the Knowledge and Reference sections.

Now, hurry up!

The Exercises

FIND THE EXERCISES designated as equal or lesser than your ability level. Review the proper exercise technique described and the photo demonstrating each exercise. Take a few minutes to try each one. Be advised, Recruit: You will bring your orders with you at least the first few times you train and each time you advance to a new level to be sure your technique is correct for every exercise. Doing your drills wrong won't get you the results you need and can get you hurt, so don't rely on your memory until you're well acquainted with every drill. Learn what you're supposed to do the right way so you develop real skills and build on them!

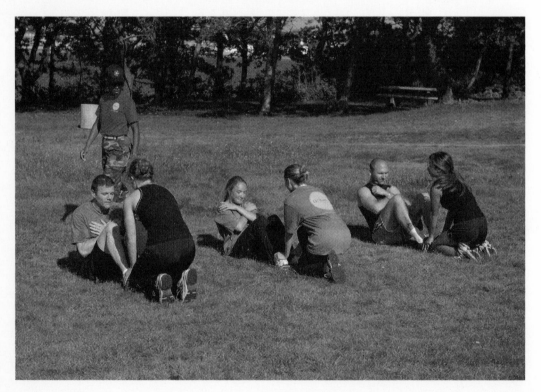

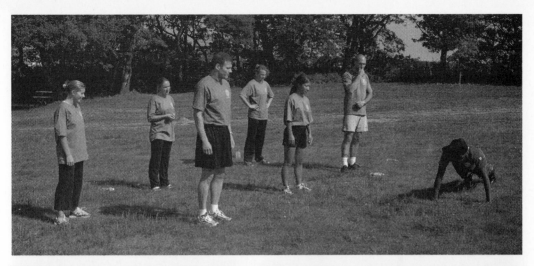

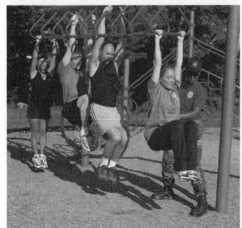

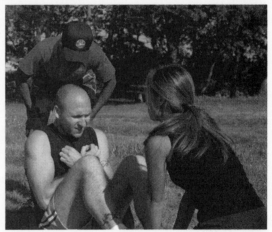

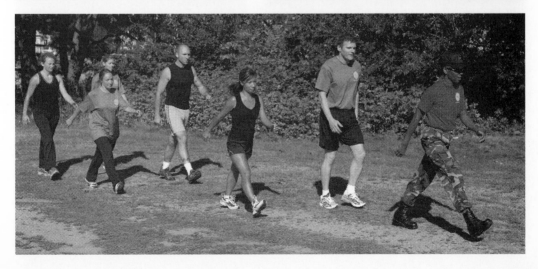

General Exercise Technique Guidelines

Proper exercise technique and good mental focus are vital to getting the most out of your training. You know now that your abs flex to curve your spine. But if you lose concentration and start rushing through any exercise, your legs, hip flexors, and lower back will all pitch in to help you move. The result? Training completed, but no real ab strength or muscular definition achieved. Pay attention and stick to strict technique.

For every one of your abdominal training exercises, the following rules apply (in addition to the specific guidance you get for each one).

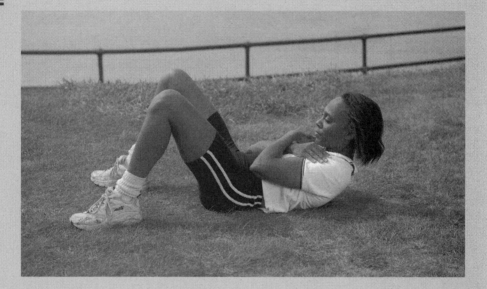

> **The job of the rectus abdominis is to curve your spine forward, so your back must bend on every repetition. If you're still doing crunches like an aerobics class refugee (back straight as a board, elbows flared out from the sides of your head), knock it off because you haven't engaged a single ab muscle fiber yet.**

> **Consciously keep your hips, lower legs, and lower back as relaxed as possible. Rock your pelvis slightly forward, roll your torso (or hips for lower body work) forward and up, and keep everything else uninvolved. Check it every 2 to 3 repetitions and readjust as necessary.**

> > >

> Start every exercise with an inhale to expand your chest and slightly flatten that ab wall. Keep breathing high in your chest as you further suck in your gut all the way down towards your hip bone. Then exhale smoothly each time you curl your torso or your hips up, depending on the exercise.

> Don't hold your breath! It creates intra-abdominal pressure that will prevent you from fully flexing your abs, and may contribute to making them stronger, but convex (rounded out; not a good look)

> For crunches and other upper-body movement drills, your shoulders and chest must leave the deck every rep. It doesn't matter how high you raise your head, you get no bonus points for tiring your neck out. Curve that spine.

> Don't rush. Except for your timed curl-ups, in which you try to complete as many as possible within a specified time limit, you will use a smooth steady flex of your abs to complete each movement. No jerking or bouncing.

Marksman

IF YOUR LEVEL IS MARKSMAN, you will use the following exercises in your training regimen.

SUPERMAN

This is a 4-count exercise; 1 rep equals two completions of the steps below.

EMPHASIS: Spinal erectors (lower back)

READY: Lie facedown on the deck with your legs straight and your arms extended straight forward.

EXERCISE!

1) Using smooth controlled movements, simultaneously raise your arms, torso, and legs a few inches off the deck.

2) Simultaneously lower your legs, arms, and torso to the Ready position.

TRAINING ADVISORY

> Do not jerk your limbs up at any point during this exercise.

> Breathe normally throughout.

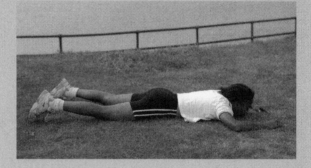

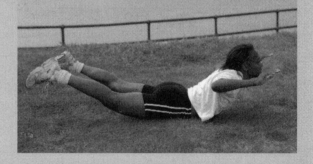

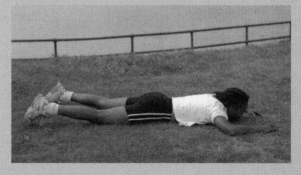

THE SWIMMER

This is a 4-count exercise; 1 rep equals two completions of the steps below.

EMPHASIS: Spinal erectors and glutes

READY: Lie facedown on the deck with your legs straight, extend your arms straight forward.

EXERCISE!

1) Using a smooth controlled movement, simultaneously raise your left arm and shoulder and your right leg a few inches off the deck.

2) Return to the Ready position.

3) Simultaneously raise your right arm and shoulder and your left leg approximately 6" off the deck

4) Return to the Ready position.

TRAINING ADVISORY

> Maintain controlled, flexing movement at all times and don't jerk your limbs up.

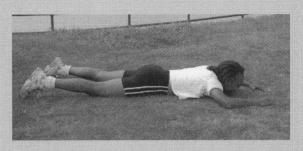
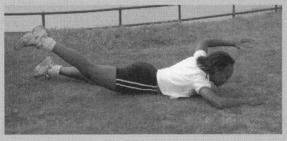
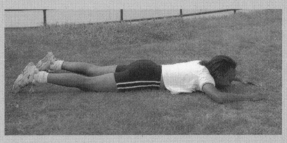
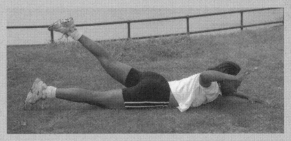
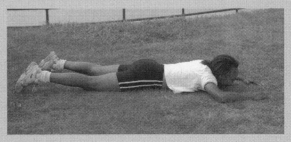

TILT-UPS, KNEES BENT

This is a 2-count exercise; 1 rep equals one completion of the steps listed below.

EMPHASIS: Rectus abdominis (abdominal muscle) lower region

READY: Lie on your back with your legs elevated and knees bent, leave your lower legs relaxed and place your hands and forearms under your hips for lumbar (lower back) support. Inhale to expand your rib cage, push your lower back (lumbar curve) flat down onto your arms, and suck your gut in toward your spine.

EXERCISE!

1) Roll your knees toward your face and flex your abs to lift your hips slightly up and off your hands.

2) Return to the Ready position

TRAINING ADVISORY

> Don't bounce! While you work to improve your abdominal strength you may only be able to raise your hips slightly off your hands. Focus on a solid flex.

> Exhale as you flex your abs and raise your hips. Flatten your abs as much as possible on every rep.

> Mentally focus on your lower abs, between your navel and just below your hip bones.

> > >

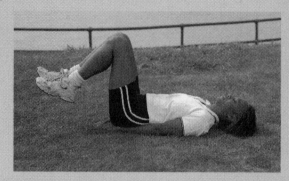
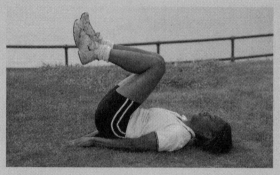
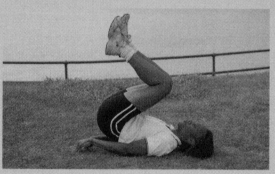
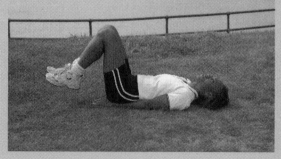

EXPERT VARIATION:
TILT-UPS, LEGS STRAIGHT

Assume the Ready position, but extend your legs straight up. Keeping your legs straight, flex your lower abs to raise your hips and lower body a few inches off your hands. Return to the Ready position.

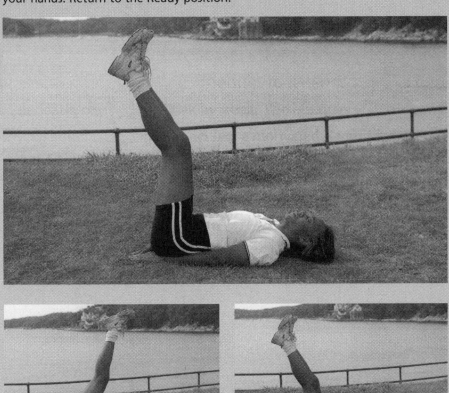

CRUNCHES

This is a 2-count exercise; 1 rep equals going once through the steps below.

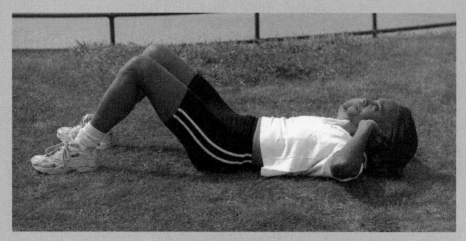

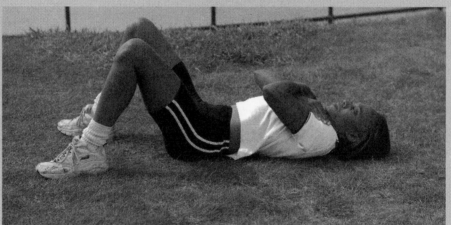

EMPHASIS: Rectus abdominis (lower region)

READY: Lie on your back with your knees bent and feet flat on the deck, place your hands either beside your ears (to provide gentle support for your head and neck), or crossed over your chest. Inhale to expand your rib cage, push your lower back flat to the deck, and suck your gut in flat toward your spine.

EXERCISE!

1) Using a controlled movement, curl your torso as far up and forward as possible toward your thighs, flexing your abs and drawing your belly in towards your spine. Exhale on your way up

> > >

2) Return to the Ready position

TRAINING ADVISORY

> Do not yank on your neck or pull your head forward at any time. If your hands are beside your ears, they are there to let your neck rest only.

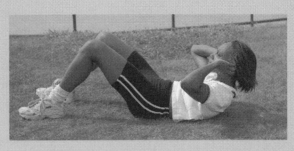

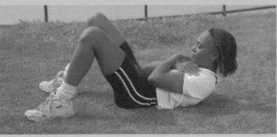

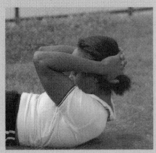

> Do not jerk your body forward. Curl up with a smooth, steady motion as you exhale.

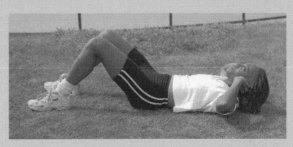

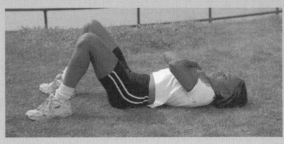

REVERSE CRUNCHES

This is a 2-count exercise; 1 rep equals one completion of the steps listed below.

EMPHASIS: Rectus abdominis (lower region)

READY: Sitting on the deck with your knees bent and feet on the deck, flex your ankles to point your toes straight up, resting your feet on your heels. Keep your knees bent so that your feet are always as close to your hips as possible. Hold your arms out straight in front of you for counterbalance. Inhale to expand your rib cage and flatten your ab wall.

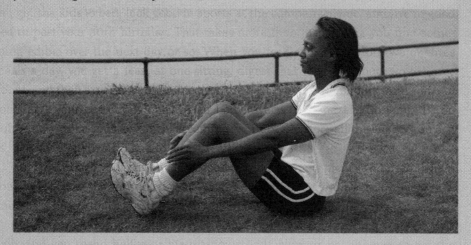

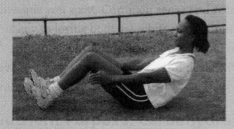
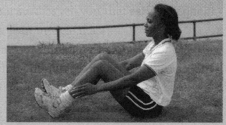

EXERCISE!

1) Using SLOW, controlled movement, keeping a curve in your lower back and exhaling on the way down, uncurl your torso backwards toward the deck, getting as low as possible without kicking your heels for balance.

2) Inhale as you return to the Ready position.

TRAINING ADVISORY

> Check your breathing at least every other rep to ensure that you're exhaling on the way down toward the deck.

> Perform each rep slowly to fully engage your lower ab fibers every time. Move too quickly and you will use your legs and back, bypassing your ab muscles completely.

> Make sure your toes stay pointed up and that your knees don't straighten out.

LEGS-UP CRUNCHES

This is a 2-count exercise; 1 rep equals one completion of the steps listed below.

EMPHASIS: Rectus abdominis (lower region)

READY: Lie on your back on the deck, raise your legs, and cross your feet at the ankles with your knees bent and lower legs relaxed. Place your hands either beside your ears (to provide gentle support for your head and neck), or crossed over your chest. Inhale to expand your rib cage, push your lower back flat to the deck, and suck your gut in flat toward your spine.

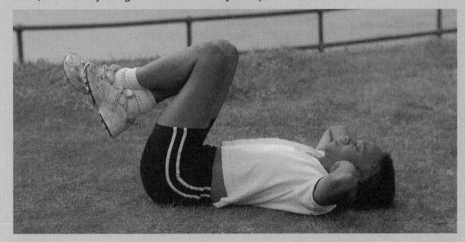

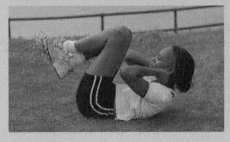
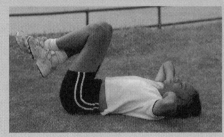

EXERCISE!

1) Curl your shoulders and torso as far up as possible toward your thighs, exhaling as you crunch up.

2) Return to the Ready position.

TRAINING ADVISORY

> You should be able to curl tighter on this exercise than in regular crunches, so roll that torso up tight.

> Leave your legs still.

LYING SIDE-BENDS

This is a 4-count exercise; 1 rep equals one completion of the steps listed below.

EMPHASIS: Rectus abdominis and obliques

READY: Lie on your back on the deck, knees bent with your feet flat and hands at your ears to gently support your head and neck.

EXERCISE!

1) Raise your shoulders very slightly, but keep your back in contact with the deck and bend your torso to the right as far as possible as though trying to touch your right shoulder to the side of your right hip.
2) Return to the Ready position.
3) Raise your shoulders again and bend your torso to the left as far as possible as though trying to touch your left shoulder to the side of your left hip.
4) Return to the Ready position.

TRAINING ADVISORY

> Mentally focus on your obliques, which run alongside your torso and waist.

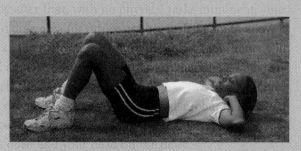
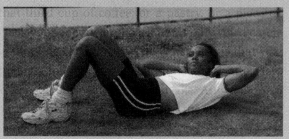
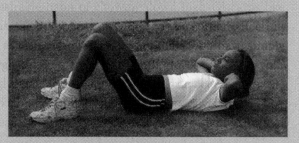
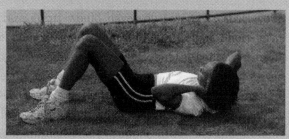
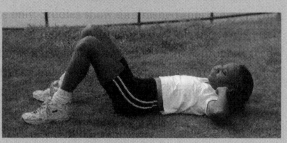

TIMED CURL-UP

This is a timed exercise. You will complete as many reps as possible within the time specified in your training plan.

EMPHASIS: Abdominal strength and endurance

READY: Lie on your back on the deck, anchor your feet under a sturdy object or have a buddy hold them. Keep your knees bent. You will focus on flexing your abs and keeping your legs, hips, and lower back as relaxed as possible.

EXERCISE!

1) When time starts, sit up by curling your torso up and forward until your elbows touch your thighs.

2) Uncurl until the bottoms of your shoulder blades (curve of the lumbar spine) touch the deck

TRAINING ADVISORY

> Don't bounce off the deck, thrust your arms forward, or raise your hips at any time to assist you in curling up.

> If you can no longer properly complete any reps, move your hips as far back as possible from your heels keeping your feet flat on the deck. Focus on the area just below your navel, and work to roll your chin toward your chest and your chest toward your hip bone.

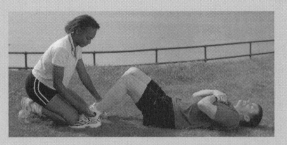
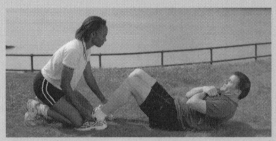
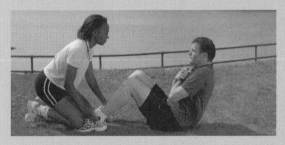
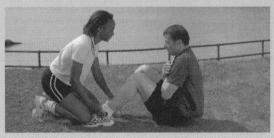
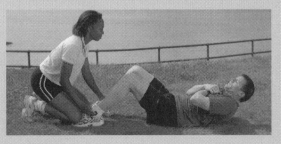

ALTERNATE LEG CRUNCHES

This is a 2-count exercise; 1 rep equals one completion of the steps listed below.

EMPHASIS: Rectus abdominis and obliques

READY: Lie on your back on the deck, knees bent with your feet flat, cross your left foot onto your right knee (your left thigh should be raised and parallel to the deck). Extend your left arm straight out to your side and rest it on the deck. Place your right hand at your ear to gently support your head and neck. Inhale to expand your rib cage.

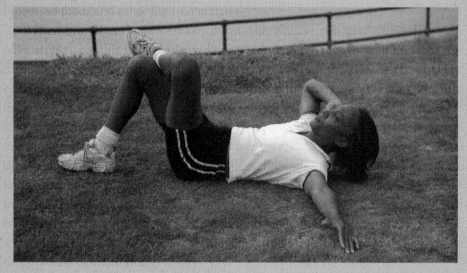

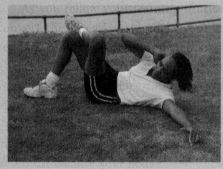

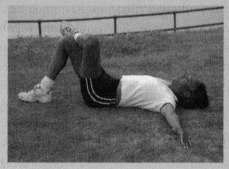

> > >

EXERCISE!

1) Raising your right shoulder, twist your torso and right shoulder as far as possible toward your left knee, exhaling as you crunch up.

2) Return to the Ready position. Once you complete the required number of reps, switch your legs and repeat for the other side.

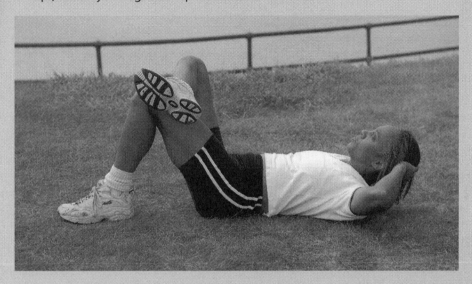

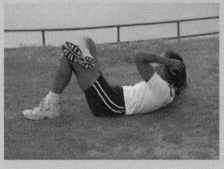
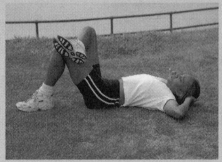

TRAINING ADVISORY

> Mentally focus on your obliques; don't move your legs.

DISTANCE RUN

This is a distance-based exercise.

EMPHASIS: Cardiovascular endurance

READY: Use a stopwatch or watch with a second hand to track your progress. Map out the distance on a track, road, or path so you will know how far you travel. Your route may be flat or may include hills for better training variation.

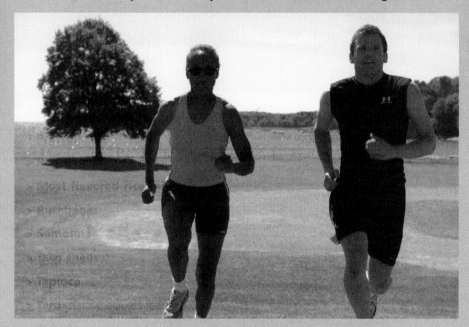

EXERCISE!

1) Run for the specified distance, maintaining an even pace and keeping your upper body—shoulders, neck, chest, and arms—relaxed. Keep your feet close to the ground with every step and keep your breathing relaxed, inhaling through your nose and exhaling through your mouth and nose.

> > >

TRAINING ADVISORY

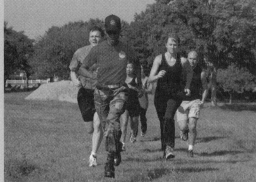

> Check your style regardless of how experienced you are at running.

> For distance running you will run heel to toe, allowing the flat surface of your heel to strike the deck first on every step and allowing your foot to roll naturally towards the ball, propelling you forward.

> Don't bounce up and down. Concentrate on smooth forward motion with minimal vertical motion and no noise.

> If you hear a slapping sound as your feet strike the deck, experience pain in your shins, or have difficulty running heel to toe, stop and schedule an appointment with a podiatrist or orthopedist (preferably a sports doctor). Chances are you have an abnormality in the arches of your feet or in your gait and require different running shoes or an orthotic device. Continuing to run incorrectly will only get you hurt—so get it checked out!

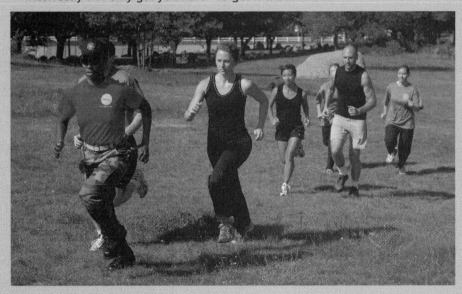

> Carry your arms low and relaxed at your sides. Don't shrug your shoulders or raise your arms.

POWER WALK (The Military "Hump")

This is a timed exercise.

EMPHASIS: Cardiovascular endurance

READY: Use a watch to track your progress. Map out the distance on a road or path so you will know how far you travel. Your route may be flat or may include hills, steps, or obstacles for better training variation.

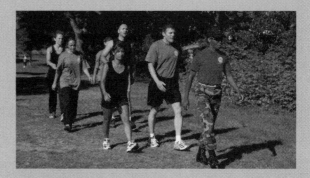

EXERCISE!

1) Taking a long, comfortable heel to toe step, every step, walk the specified distance within the specified time limit.

TRAINING ADVISORY

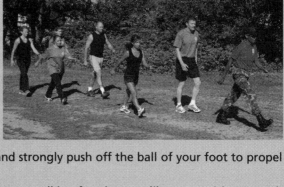

> Extend your legs with each step, so that your heel strikes the deck first, and strongly push off the ball of your foot to propel your body forward.

> Your technique should have you walking fast, but not like competitive "speed walking" in which individuals walk as fast as possible but using short steps— these are the folks who look like cartoons in fast-motion snapping their knees sharply back on every step. Extend your stride and use all the muscles in your upper legs!

EXPERT VARIATION:

Strap on a backpack filled with books, clothing, and shoes, or sandbags for a load of 30 to 70 pounds to increase your difficulty level.

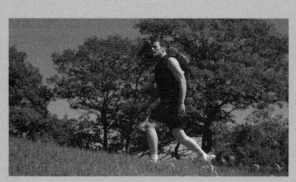

INTERVAL SPRINTS

This is a distance and perceived effort based exercise.

EMPHASIS: Cardiovascular endurance

READY: Use a stopwatch or a watch with a second hand to track your progress. Map out the distance on a track, road, or path. You will need to mark landmarks about every 25 yards. Your route should be flat. NOTE: An average high school or college track circling a football field is ¼-mile around, lines on the field are marked every ten yards; an average indoor track is ⅛-mile around; an average city block is 100 to 140 yards. On city streets, use street lights and utility poles as landmarks. In the suburbs, use mailboxes and street lights as landmarks.

EXERCISE!

1) Placing all of your weight on the balls of your feet and never allowing your heels to strike the deck, run the specified distance at the exertion level prescribed (based on how you feel), using a pumping action with your arms and taking comfortably long steps with each foot.

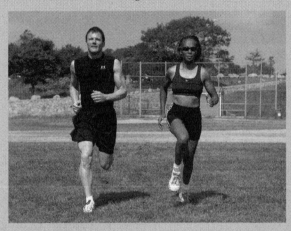

TRAINING ADVISORY

> Your training plan will list the required number of reps and pacing for each sprint.

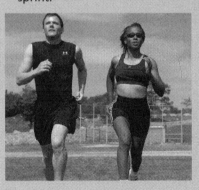

> Keep your chest and torso up and forward; focus on exploding off the start line and through every step from start to finish.

> If you have a buddy, use each other for pacing (without getting ruthlessly competitive or held back by your buddy's pace and skill level).

Sharpshooter

IF YOUR LEVEL IS SHARPSHOOTER, you will use the following exercises in addition to the Marksman exercises for your training.

FLUTTER KICKS

This is a 4-count exercise; 1 rep equals one completion of the steps listed below.

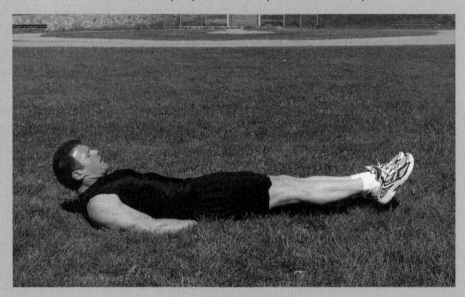

EMPHASIS: Rectus abdominis (lower region)

READY: Lie flat on your back on the deck, legs out straight, hands placed under your lower back and hips for lumbar support. Inhale high in your chest to expand your rib cage, press your lower back flat down onto your arms, and raise both legs off the deck to your Ground-Zero Estimate (the lowest point where you can keep the arch out of your back). Keep your knees slightly bent.

EXERCISE!

1) Raise your left leg 2 to 3" up.

2) Simultaneously lower your left leg to the Ready position and raise your right leg 2 to 3".

> > >

3) Simultaneously lower your right leg to the Ready position and raise your left leg 2 to 3"

4) Simultaneously lower your left leg and raise your right leg.

TRAINING ADVISORY

> Keep your chest and rib cage high and breathe comfortably.

> Focus lower on your ab wall throughout the exercise and keep your knees slightly bent to avoid fatiguing the legs.

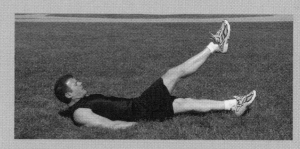

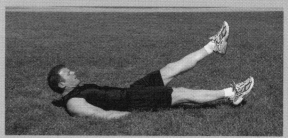

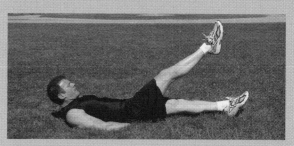

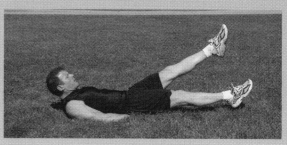

FOUR-COUNT CRUNCHES

Obviously, this is a 4-count exercise; 1 rep equals one completion of the steps listed below.

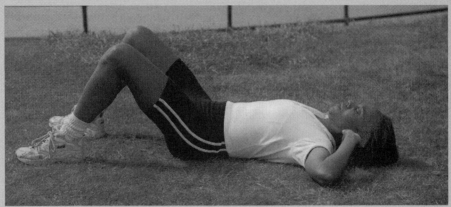

EMPHASIS: Rectus abdominis

READY: Lie on your back on the deck, knees bent, feet flat with your arms either at your ears to gently support your head and neck or across your chest. Inhale high in your chest to expand your rib cage and push your back flat to the deck.

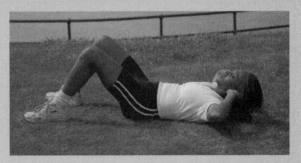

EXERCISE!

1) Focusing on your upper ab fibers only, curl your shoulders and chest up approximately 3" off the deck.

2) Focusing on your upper and mid-torso ab fibers, continue curling your shoulders and chest about 2" farther forward.

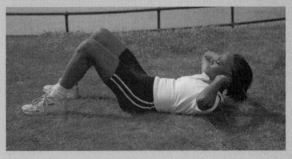

> > >

3) Focusing on your entire abdominal wall (sucking your lower gut in toward your spine), continue curling your torso as far up and forward as possible.

4) Return to the Ready position.

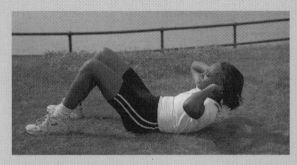

TRAINING ADVISORY

> Don't let gravity take over when returning to the Ready position; use control.

> Exhale steadily through each of the upward movements.

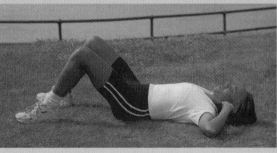

> Make each of the three upward movements distinct, with a slight pause after each.

> Keep your back flat and abs sucked in during the upward crunches.

SIX-COUNT CRUNCHES

One rep equals one completion of the steps listed below. The exercise begins the same as the 4-count crunch and adds work for the obliques at the end of each rep.

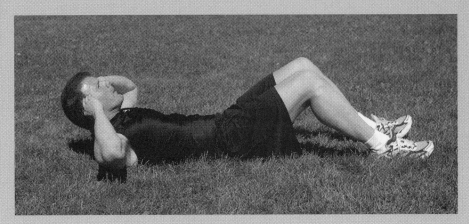

EMPHASIS: Rectus abdominis, external obliques

READY: Lie on your back on the deck, knees bent, feet flat with your arms either at your ears to gently support your head and neck or crossed across your chest. Inhale high in your chest to expand your rib cage and push your lower back flat to the deck.

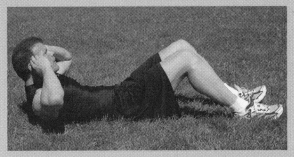

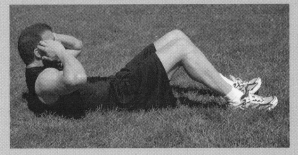

EXERCISE!

1) Focusing on your upper ab fibers, curl your shoulders and chest up approximately 3" off the deck.

2) Focusing on your upper and mid-torso ab fibers, continue curling your shoulders and chest about 2" farther up.

3) Focusing on your entire abdominal wall (sucking in your lower gut), continue curling your torso as far up and forward as possible.

> > >

4) Still in the torso forward position of count 3, twist your right shoulder toward your left thigh by flexing your obliques.

5) Still in the torso forward position, twist your left shoulder toward your right thigh, by flexing your obliques.

6) Return to the Ready position.

TRAINING ADVISORY

> Exhale steadily through all 5 crunching movements.

> Make each crunching/twisting movement distinct with a slight pause after each.

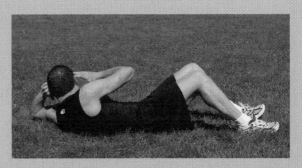

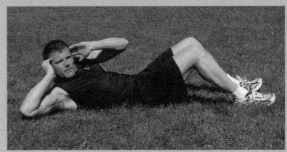

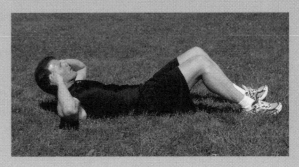

TILT-UPS, STRAIGHT LEGS

This is a 2-count exercise; 1 rep equals one completion of the steps listed below.

EMPHASIS: Rectus abdominis

READY: Lie on your back on the deck with legs extended straight up (perpendicular to the deck) leaving a slight bend in the knees. Place your hands and forearms under your lower back and hips for lumbar support and inhale high in your chest to expand your rib cage.

EXERCISE!

1) Without bouncing, flex your abs to lift your hips off your hands.

2) Return to the READY position.

TRAINING ADVISORY

> Don't BOUNCE! Focus on a smooth solid flex with a brief pause in the "up" position.

> Exhale as you raise your hips and suck in your gut (especially lower down toward your hip bone)

> Mentally focus on those lower ab fibers.

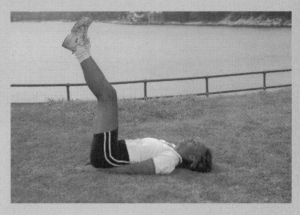

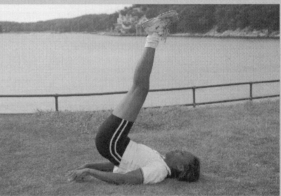

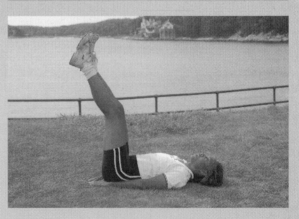

HILL TRAINING

This is a rep-based exercise that will be included with Distance Run on some days.

EMPHASIS: Cardiovascular strength

READY: Locate a path or road that incorporates a hill or series of short hills. If your hills are very steep or long, you can either reduce the specified number of reps until your endurance improves, or accept the tougher challenge if you are already conditioned. If you have no hills near you, you can substitute stair running to get similar benefits.

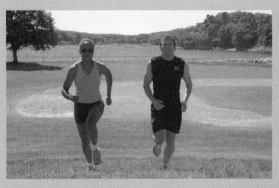

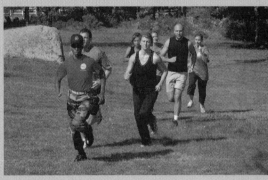

EXERCISE!

1) Begin at the bottom of the hill and run up at the specified pace, focusing on keeping your abs tight, crunching your torso slightly forward, and flexing your quads.

2) Return to the bottom of the hill at the specified recovery pace, focusing on keeping your back relaxed and controlling your speed.

3) Repeat for the prescribed number of reps.

TRAINING ADVISORY

> Don't let gravity take over on your recovery run down the hill. You must control your body all the way down to avoid losing control of your pace.

> Maintain the same running style prescribed for distance running under Marksman exercises.

Expert

IF YOUR LEVEL IS EXPERT, you will use the following exercises in addition to the Marksman and Sharpshooter exercises for your training.

TOTAL-BODY CRUNCHES

This is a 2-count exercise; 1 rep equals one completion of the steps listed below.

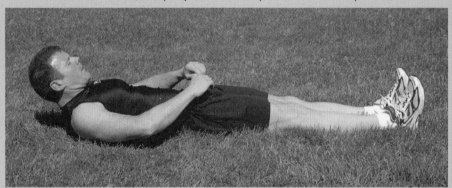

EMPHASIS: Rectus abdominis
READY: Lie on your back with legs straight (knees slightly bent) and arms either across your chest or placed at your ears to gently support your head and neck. Inhale high in your chest to expand your rib cage.
EXERCISE!

1) Pushing your hips down to the deck and sucking your gut in toward your spine, simultaneously crunch your torso forward toward your hip bone and tuck your knees up toward your chest. Tuck up as tightly as possible without jerking.

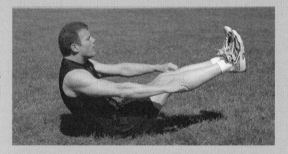

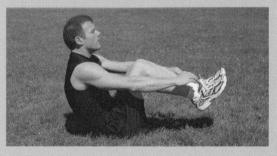

> > >

2) Return to the READY position, only allowing your heels to touch the deck briefly before repeating for the specified number of reps.

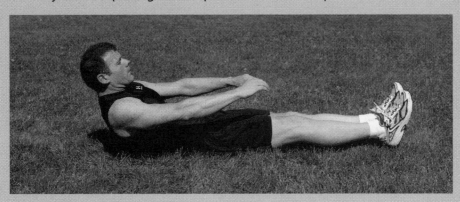

TRAINING ADVISORY

> Don't jerk your body up.
> Exhale as you crunch your whole body up.

SINGLE-LEG CRUNCHES

This is a 2-count exercise; 1 rep equals one completion of the steps listed below.

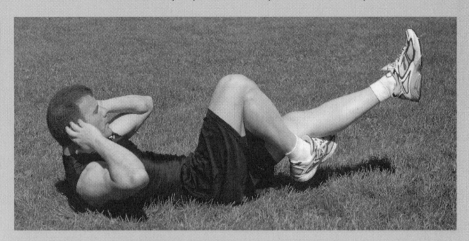

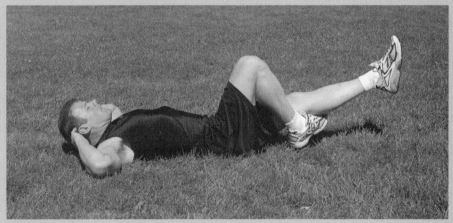

EMPHASIS: Rectus abdominis

READY: Lie on your back with legs straight, raise your left leg 6 to 8" off the deck. Hook your right foot under your left calf to help support your straight leg. Place your arms across your chest or place your hands at your ears to gently support your head and neck. Inhale high in your chest to expand your rib cage and press your lower back (lumbar curve) down toward the deck.

EXERCISE!

1) Pushing your lower back flat to the deck and your abs flat to your back, curl your shoulders and chest as far toward your hip bone as possible.

2) Uncurl your torso to return to the READY position.

> > >

3) Halfway through the required number of reps, switch your legs (extend the other leg) and complete the reps.

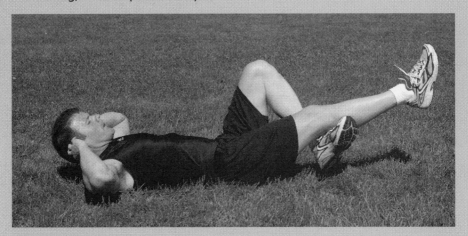

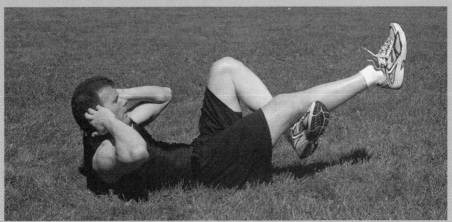

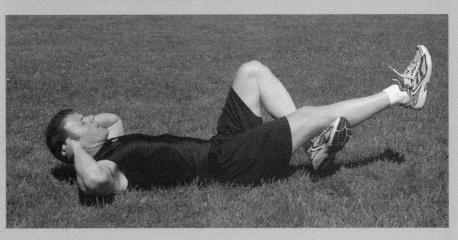

V-SITS, KNEES BENT

This is a 2-count exercise; 1 rep equals one completion of the steps listed below.

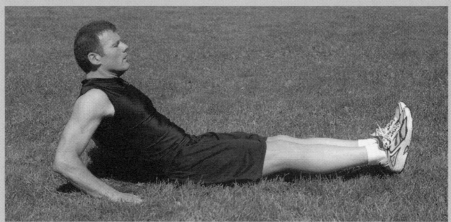

EMPHASIS: Rectus abdominis

READY: Sit on the deck balanced on your buttocks with your legs extended in front of you, feet resting on their heels on the deck. Lean your torso back to about 45 degrees from the deck with your hands lightly touching the deck beside your hips or, for added difficulty, with your arms extended out straight for counterbalance.

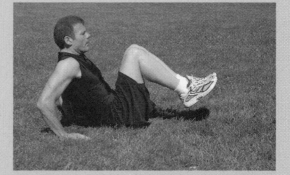

EXERCISE!

1) Simultaneously, tuck your knees up into your chest and raise your torso up and forward toward your thighs

2) Lower both torso and legs to the ready position.

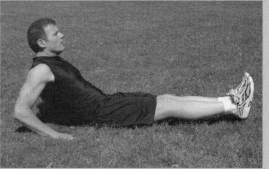

TRAINING ADVISORY

> Maintain your balance. It will take practice until you find the point at which you can remain balanced both while outstretched and while crunching up.

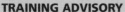

V-SITS, LEGS STRAIGHT

This is a 2-count exercise; 1 rep equals one completion of the steps listed below.

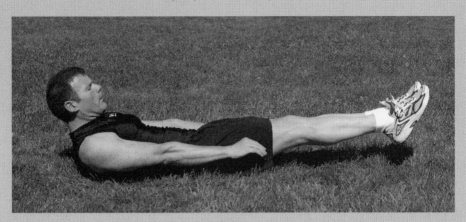

EMPHASIS: Rectus abdominis

READY: Sit on the deck balanced on your buttocks with your legs extended in front of you, feet resting on their heels on the deck. Lean your torso back to about 45 degrees from the deck with with your hands lightly touching the deck beside your hips or, for added difficulty, with your arms extended out straight for counterbalance.

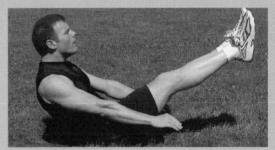

EXERCISE!

1) Simultaneously, lift your legs (keeping them straight) and raise your torso up and forward toward your legs as though trying to touch your chest to your shins

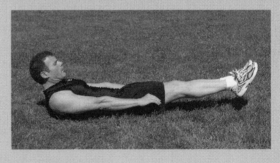

2) Lower both torso and legs to the ready position.

TRAINING ADVISORY

> Maintain your balance. It will take practice until you find the point at which you can remain balanced both while outstretched and while crunching up.

> Exhale as you crunch your whole body up.

> > >

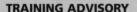

VARIATION:
BENCH V-SITS (Knees Bent or Legs Straight)

Begin the exercise by sitting at the edge of a bench, balanced on your buttocks, with your torso leaning back about 45 degrees and your hands placed behind your back on the bench for balance. Your legs will hang over the front edge of the bench allowing you to fully stretch your ab wall each time you lower your legs to the Ready position. Perform the exercise the same as above for either Knees Bent or Legs Straight variations.

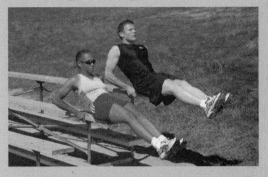

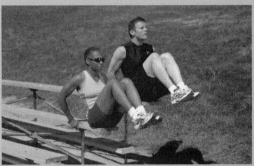

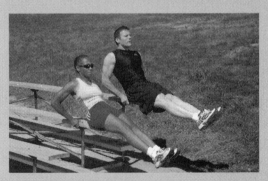

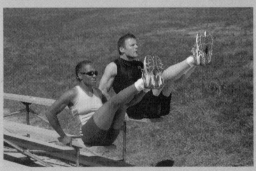

SIDE V-RAISES

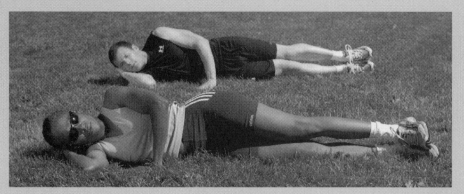

This is a 2-count exercise; 1 rep equals one completion of the steps listed below.

EMPHASIS: Rectus abdominis, external obliques

READY: Lie on the deck on your right side with legs extended, left leg on top of the right and recline on the right side of your torso. Keep your right arm comfortably placed forward of your torso and bend your left arm across your torso with the palm of your hand resting on the deck.

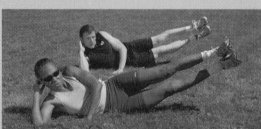

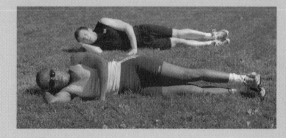

EXERCISE!

1) Simultaneously raise both legs and your torso as though trying to touch your left shoulder to your left hip.

2) Lower torso and legs to the Ready position.

3) Repeat for the specified number of reps, then repeat on the other side.

TRAINING ADVISORY

> Maintain your balance. It will take practice until you find the point at which you can remain balanced while crunching up.

> Do not push up with the arm that's crossed over your torso; it's there for balance only

> You will only be able to rise up a few inches at your torso. Do not jerk your body or pull excessively with your legs. If you are getting major air off the deck, you're pulling with your hip flexor and not engaging your obliques. Focus on the small muscles at your side.

HANGING LEG RAISES, KNEES BENT

This is a 2-count exercise requiring a pull-up bar or other anchored overhead bar; 1 rep equals one completion of the steps listed below.

EMPHASIS: Rectus abdominis, external obliques

READY: Take an overhand grip on a pull-up bar and fully extend your arms so that you hang straight down from the bar. Cross your legs at the ankles. Inhale high in your chest to expand your rib cage.

EXERCISE!

1) Tuck your knees up toward your chest as high as possible, allowing your hips to roll forward

2) Return to the Ready position.

TRAINING ADVISORY

> Keep your body from swinging by keeping your rib cage high and your abs tight as your legs descend.

> DON'T jerk your body up. Raise your knees only as high as your abs can flex them.

> Exhale as you roll your lower body up.

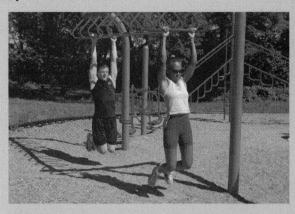

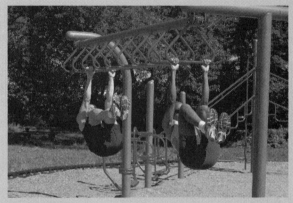

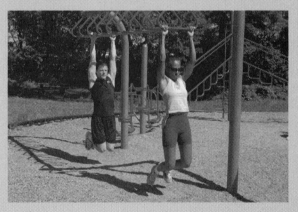

> > >

VARIATION:
HANGING LEG RAISES (Straight Leg)

Without crossing your ankles and leaving your legs extended, flex your lower abs to raise your legs 90 degrees until they are straight out in front of your body. Return to the Ready position.

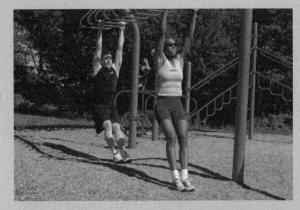

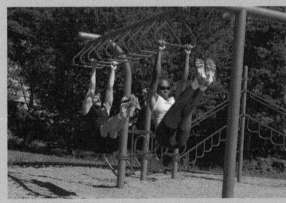

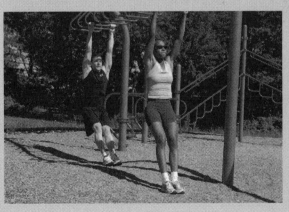

knowledge

This section contains the Briefings to review now and to then read in depth, one by one, week by week. The briefings will teach you how you should train, eat, and act like a motivated Recruit in order to complete the *Boot Camp Abs* mission. Think! Analyze! Review! Reason! You will fuel for your physical work with balanced nutrition from quality sources and, if necessary, with proven supplements. Armed with this knowledge, you'll be prepared to succeed.

BRIEFING #1
Feeding Frequency and Nutrient Purpose: Carbohydrates

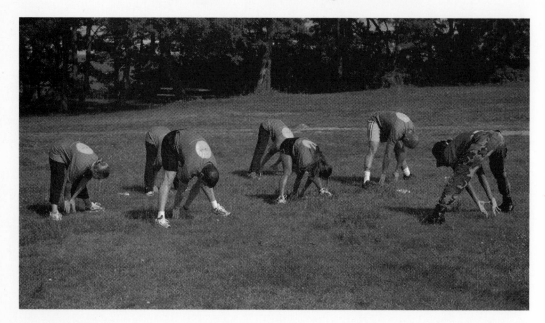

WHETHER YOUR OBJECTIVES involve fat loss, muscle gain, performance improvement, or all three, what you put in your mouth—and when—will significantly impact your progress. Your body wants to use food for the right purposes: carbs and fats for energy; proteins for muscle-building and body repair. Regardless of what chow time looks like for you, whether elegant dinners or snacks wrapped in paper, it's all just fuel to your body. The questions remain: Are you filling the tank on a schedule that keeps the machine running well and are you putting premium fuel in the tank?

Eat Often

If you're like most recruits I've seen, you've fallen into one of three bad nutrition habits:

1) **Skipping meals. Either you're desperate to lose weight and you thought starving would be a good method, or you've surrendered your health and performance to your busy schedule.**

2) **Still eating old-school ("three squares" a day). You belly up to the buffet table at six-hour intervals, get really tired a few hours after eating, and become addicted to coffee, soda, or chocolate for energy boosts.**

3) **Eating frequently but not enough: In your misguided effort to trim down or stay thin, you consume only minuscule portions of low-calorie and empty-calorie foods. You're in a permanent state of starvation.**

To begin to correct your bad habits, you will have to concentrate on eating often enough and getting quality nutrients every time you eat.

Direct Order #1:

Effective immediately, you will put quality food in your mouth every three to four hours from Reveille to Taps every day with your last meal no more than three hours before Lights Out. To be clear: that's at least four to six small meals every day, possibly more depending on how long you're awake.

I can already hear some of you sounding off without permission. You just aren't hungry that often, and you've been told that you shouldn't eat if you're not hungry. Pay attention, Recruit. If you don't get hungry every four hours—at maximum—it means your body has stopped sending regular hunger signals because you've eaten so badly for so long. When your body doesn't get the fuel it needs (like when you starve yourself on extremely low-calorie or monotonous diets), you will simply lose your appetite within two to four days. Think of it this way: If you kept submitting requests that always got denied, wouldn't you give up and turn your energy to other things? Yes, and your body stopped submitting requests for an efficient eating schedule soon after your mom stopped planning your snack times. Meanwhile, your metabolism has slowed to a snail's pace to keep you alive on that tiny bit of energy from your erratic feedings. So yes, you may have to force yourself to follow a reasonable eating schedule for about four or five days and then your system should wake up and start requesting food as frequently as it should.

"But I don't eat very much now," you're thinking, "and if I'm trying to lose weight or stay trim, why do you want me to eat more?"

If you consistently eat far less or less often than what you truly need to perform well, your body prepares for the day when there won't be any food at all. It works to keep the fat storage area full so you can survive when that happens. Give it a steady supply of appropriate fuel, however, and it learns that there is no need to panic—it opens up the fat storage area and begins to burn.

Your body is programmed to expect either feast or famine; you learned that while roaming the plains a few millenia ago. A good day meant an animal kill or the successful gathering of fruits and berries so you could eat for a few hours. A bad day meant, "Keep walking because there's nothing to eat here." Under those circumstances, your mission was simple: Just keep the brain and vital organs functioning. Stay alive. Survive!

Fast-forward several thousand years. Now you need to get the kids to school, make sound business decisions, work hard at your job eight to sixteen hours a day, battle traffic, pick up the dry cleaning, get the kids from school, pay bills, feed the cat, get the kids to bed, look good in shorts at the company picnic, and live in good health past your 30th birthday. That takes more than just hoping you find something edible over the next day or so. When you feed sporadically on two or three meals a day, you get a feast at one sitting, digest that food in about two to three hours, and then experience a famine over the next two to seven hours. And some of you starve yourselves even longer. Your body reverts to Stone Age thinking: If you don't know when your next meal is coming, you'd better store all the energy you can as body fat to stay warm and to keep breathing.

To get through your day and look good at that company picnic, you need to help your body make the most of the fuel it gets. When you ate dinner at about 1900 hours last night (that's 7 P.M., Recruit), skipped breakfast this morning, and didn't go to chow again until noon today, you just went on a seventeen-hour fast! Do that daily and you spend half your life malnourished, which is not the way to get the physique you want. Common sense and recent studies tell you that eating frequently is key to losing body fat while maintaining lean muscle mass.

Still not convinced, Recruit? Then put on your thinking cap and start by getting squared away on how your system deals with its preferred energy source, carbohydrates.

Nutrient Purpose: Carbohydrates

Recall your last meal, which I'm sure was a tasty, nutritionally balanced selection of complex carbohydrates, quality protein, minimal fats, and some fiber. Your digestive system wakes up to start processing the fuel. Your small intestines release enzymes for breaking the nutrients down to their usable forms. For immediate energy, it breaks down the carbohydrates.

Carbs provide your body's primary energy source, and they're present to some degree in nearly everything you'll eat on a normal diet. Your digestive enzymes get right to work breaking the carbs down. Expecting the fuel shipment, your pancreas starts releasing insulin to deliver it to your muscles and brain which need it to function. Now pay attention, because the insulin release is high priority.

DIAGRAM 1

Glucose Breakdown/Insulin Transport
Dietary carbohydrate (bread, rice, pasta, etc.)

Converted to glucose in small intestine ⟳ Insulin release from pancreas

⟱

Muscle glycogen ⟲ Glucose transported through blood ⟳ Liver glycogen

Adipose tissue ⟱ Excreted in urine
(fat deposits)

⟱

Other tissues
(for energy)

All carbohydrates are made of carbon, oxygen, and hydrogen and all are broken down to glucose before travelling through the bloodstream (what we call "blood sugar") to the appropriate destination: a short-term holding area for energy, or long-term storage as body fat.

What goes where?

Well, that depends on what kind of carbs you ate and what activity is next on your agenda. Carbs are properly categorized according to their glycemic index (GI) which is a relative measure of how quickly a particular food is broken down to that simplest form (glucose, remember?). The lower the GI, the more slowly the carbs break down, giving you time to burn the fuel as it comes in. High GI carbs are the ones for which you need to watch out. These foods break down to glucose very quickly and are rapidly introduced into the bloodstream.

What's the big deal?

Imagine your brain getting word that a huge fuel shipment (glucose) is incoming and requires processing. Glucose pours into your bloodstream from that Thanksgiving-sized meal of pasta, corn on the cob, and breadsticks you just inhaled, and the pancreas sends a carrier load of insulin to transport it to your brain and nervous system, muscles, and liver for energy and normal functioning. Blood sugar is streaming into your system double time, but there's a hitch...

Chances are you aren't running a marathon in the next few hours, so there's no immediate use for that much fuel. You're experiencing hyperglycemia—your blood sugar level is much higher than necessary. You're full, energized, cheerful, good to go—for about a half hour. Shortly after that, with no physical tasks imminent, your body sends the excess fuel to a holding area for future use because it cannot allow it to keep circulating. That means all the fuel you can't burn in the next few hours will be converted to fat and stored in adipose tissue (check your love handles). That carrier load of insulin quickly escorts the excess glucose out of your bloodstream and into storage. Your energy level drops. You're tired, weak, and probably in a bad mood. Your condition has changed to hypoglycemia, and there's barely enough fuel left circulating to keep your eyes open and your head off the desk.

Here's where you reach for that third cup of coffee, or a pastry, or a piece of chocolate, or a soda—anything to pick your energy level back up. If only you'd eaten like you have good sense, you'd be thinking clearly now. The worst part is that you keep repeating the cycle—hyperglycemia followed by hypoglycemia—day after day, week after week trying to balance your blood sugar and stay awake. And you don't burn the stored fat because your body is now trained to keep it for the Great Famine you hint at during those seventeen hour mini-fasts.

If you've developed an undesirable habit of chowing down high-GI carbs like sugars and overprocesssed grains, then pay close attention to your orders, Recruit. You are not "addicted" to carbs as claimed by moronic fad diets. You have simply fallen prey to the cycle of hyperglycemia (a sugar rush with glucose flooding your bloodstream), followed by hypoglycemia (the energy plummet that occurs when the fuel glut has to be whisked off to storage), followed by more hyperglycemia (as you try to wake up), and so on. To break the cycle, you will choose better-quality fuel and feed yourself at regular intervals.

The current low-carb diet craze gurus would have you severely restrict your intake of the body's preferred fuel on a misguided quest to lose weight. Short-term studies have found that people do lose weight on these diets; but the consensus from comparing studies is that the weight loss comes from reducing total calories over longer periods of time, not from reducing the carbs. But there are other problems that come with sharply reducing carb intake. Although your muscles can learn to function at substandard levels by retrieving minuscule energy supplies from fats and protein, your brain cannot; it runs on carbs only. Studies show diminished short-term memory performance (not to mention worse moods) with low-blood glucose levels after insufficient carbohydrate intake of only a few hours compared to those properly feeding their brains. To be fair, since fats can only be processed for energy in the presence of oxygen, the bodies of serious endurance athletes can make efficient use of fats for fuel. Sedentary folks and recreational athletes, however, will find themselves markedly short of energy and mental focus, and therefore, ultimately, far short of desirable

DIAGRAM 2

Getting the Energy You Need

While the body can get energy from any of the three major nutrients, carbohydrates and fats are the primary sources.

Protein   Carbohydrate   Fat

blood glucose ⮕ ATP
(high energy compound)

amino acids   Acetyl CoA   fatty acids

KREBS cycle

A series of reactions in which hydrogen and electrons
are used to form the high-energy compound ATP used for energy to move

ATP

(adenosine triphosphate = PPP)

When you need to move

Demand for Energy

Muscles

glycogen glucose liver
(through bloodstream)

small amount of ATP
for energy + creatine phosphate

One P is broken off, generating energy
Energy
PP ⮕ P1

P + P +creatine phosphate

PPP(ATP)   movement (5-6 seconds)   More movement
+ creatine   required

physiques and performance—even if the bodies are slightly smaller.

If you're overdoing the carbs, you will correct your habits by making better choices and not by eliminating the most efficient fuel source from your diet. Use your brain!

Most people simply need to put quality fuel in the tank and then watch that fuel work efficiently. Starting today, you will consume frequent servings of low-GI carbs—foods that break down relatively slowly in your body. By doing so, you will help your body resist, and ultimately stop, its cravings for smorgasbords of sugars, processed foods and other high-GI carbs.

When low-GI carbs are broken down, the glucose still gets shipped to your bloodstream, but this time the deliveries are slow enough that you can burn the fuel through your regular daily activities and training. Some of the glucose gets converted to glycogen, the main form that your body uses for energy, and is stored in your muscles and in your liver. To use the glycogen for energy, your body converts it to adenosine triphosphate (ATP), which is required for every single movement you make, including turning these pages. Small amounts of glycogen are converted at a time, and your muscles store these small amounts of ATP and another fuel form known as phosphocreatine (PC) to let you continue flexing your muscles for a short time. All in all, if you had to rely on only the ATP-PC stored in your muscles, you'd be able to move very quickly or very powerfully—for about five seconds. Think hard, you probably need to exercise for a little longer than that, so there must be more to this process, right? Right.

As you follow your training routine and complete your daily activities, you convert the glycogen stored in your muscles into more ATP. Your body then sends a request for reinforcements: "more glycogen, please." You make more glycogen from the small amount of glucose circulating in your blood, and then your liver releases some of its glucose stores back into the bloodstream to keep the process moving.

You should start to see why you always need a small, but steady supply of incoming glucose. The bloodstream cannot keep circulating a large quantity of this fuel. You must balance your body's need to burn its preferred fuel for brain and muscle activity without consuming so much, at one sitting or overall, that you leave excess to be stored as body fat.

To make sure you always have the energy to train hard, you must feed your muscles a steady supply of glycogen. You will keep your insulin deliveries small and well-timed, so you never feel the plummet that always follows a huge release. When you plunge into hypoglycemia, you cannot produce more glycogen for many hours because all the fuel has been shipped to storage and your body cannot open that warehouse for several hours. But consistently small, steady insulin deliveries mean that your muscles get to start each training session full of all the glycogen they can hold. And your body keeps up with your general energy demands, including moderate training activities, because you maintain constant levels of fuel between training sessions and other demanding life activities.

Direct Order #2:

Each of your small, daily meals, will include quality, low-GI carbs that get converted to glucose relatively slowly.

Listed below are some better-quality, low-GI carbs you should advance toward, and some less preferable, high-GI carbs from which you should retreat. You will inspect your cabinets, pantry, refrigerator, and restaurant menus and make the necessary adjustments.

BE ADVISED: Here and in later Briefings, the command to **RETREAT** from certain foods does not necessarily mean "abandon ship!" unless your objectives include elite-level training or competitive sports performance, you can splurge occasionally on the foods in the **RETREAT** list. Just limit your extravagances to very small servings or one to two "feasts" a month and you'll pass muster.

RETREAT FROM

> **Most sugars** (look for all forms on labels and disregard deceptions like "all-natural" or "organic"—it's still sugar, Recruit, get rid of it!)

> **Glucose**

> **Sucrose**

> **High-fructose corn syrup**

> **Maltose**

> **Dextrose**

> **Brown sugar**

> **Molasses**

> **Breadfruit**

> **Candy**

> **Cornmeal**

> **Doughnuts**

> **Gnocchi**

> **Green gram dal**

> **Ice cream and frozen yogurt** (see real dairy substitutes under Milk sugar in the "Advance Toward" column)

> **Jowar flour** (sweet white sorghum; gluten-free)

> **Low-fiber cereal** (such as cornflakes, puffed rice or wheat, sugar-topped brands)

> **Packaged, processed macaroni and cheese**

> **Mango**

> **Millet**

> **Most crackers** (read the ingredients to find ones that might be acceptable)

> **Parsnips**

> **Pastries**

> **Pretzels**

> **Ragi** (millet farmed in Malaysia and India)

> **Most flavored rice cakes**

> **Rutabagas**

> **Semolina**

> **Taco shells**

> **Tapioca**

> **Taro** (starchy, edible tuber)

> **Tofu frozen desserts** (that are sweetened with sugar)

> **Varagu** (millet farmed in Malaysia and India)

> **White bread and white flour products** (including pasta, bagels, white pita)

> **White rice**

ADVANCE TOWARD

> **Fructose** (the kind that occurs naturally in fruits and crystalline pure fructose that may appear in some quality sports drinks)

> **Products sweetened by pure fruit juice** (with no added processed sugar)

> **Pure fruit juices**

> **Apples**

> **Apricots**

> **Bananas**

> **Barley**

> **Brown rice**

> **Brown rice syrup sweetened products** (but don't go overboard)

> **Buckwheat pancakes**

> **Cherries** (fresh ones, not those found floating in syrup!)

> **Chickpeas**

> **Dried beans**

> **Gram dal or chana dal** (sweet lentils, relative to the chickpea)

> **Grapes**

> **Grapefruit**

> **High-fiber cereal** (such as Cream of Wheat®, bran flakes, Grapenuts®, Kashi Go Lean® , etc.)

> **Hominy**

> **Kidney beans**

> **Lentils**

> **Lungjow bean thread**

> **Milk sugar** (lactose, choose fat-free milk, chocolate milk, no-sugar-added ice cream)

> **New potatoes**

> **Oats and oatmeal** (yes, even a few no-sugar oatmeal cookies in moderation)

> **Oranges**

> **Peaches**

> **Peanuts** (but watch for the fat, more on that later)

> **Pears**

> **Plums**

> **Rajmah**

> **Rye**

> **Soybeans**

> **Strawberries**

> **Sweet potatoes**

> **Vitari**

> **Whole wheat breads and pasta** (but avoid products with added sugar; read the labels)

NOTE: The following foods have a higher GI, but should be included because they contain many important vitamins and other nutrients. Besides, you don't know too many obese folks who blame their problem on too much watermelon!

> **Cantaloupe**

> **Pineapple**

> **Watermelon**

The Carb Cousin: Fiber

What's the official word on fiber? It's good for you, so get some.

Fiber is found in plant foods and belongs in the carb family. Unlike other nutrients, fiber doesn't actually get digested. It resists being broken down by your digestive enzymes, and that's the secret of its success at keeping your cholesterol levels in check, reducing and stabilizing your blood sugar levels. Essentially, fiber is a speed bump keeping the traffic of digestion moving slowly enough that you have a chance to use the fuel and remove waste efficiently, without back-ups.

When you included a little bran in your morning cereal and had that sandwich on whole wheat bread, the fiber content helped slow down the conversion of carbs to glucose. Even high-GI carbs and fats moved more slowly through your digestive system. You were better able to burn the fuel as it was delivered instead of storing it as body fat, so fiber helped with your fat reduction efforts. By keeping the cholesterol traffic in check, fiber helped avoid artery blockages. And by helping you to move waste from your colon without straining, fiber helped prevent colon cancer, diverticulitis, hernias, and varicose veins. Sound like a good idea? Yes, make sure you get some daily.

Direct Order #3:

Include high-fiber foods to help you process your fuel efficiently, provide backup in your battle against excess body fat, and keep your bowel movements regular (you should have to "go" at least once a day and you shouldn't need to spend more than two to three minutes in there).

Here are the high-fiber food sources you should **ADVANCE TOWARD**. Get some today!

ADVANCE TOWARD

> **Fruits with their peel**

> **Apples**

> **Blackberries**

> **Cherries** (fresh ones, not those found in syrup!)

> **Dried apricots, dates, figs**

> **Nectarines**

> **Oranges**

> **Peaches**

> **Pears**

> **Prunes**

> **Raisins**

> **Raspberries**

> **Strawberries**

> **Grains and Breads**

> **Corn**

> **Popcorn** (plain)

> **Rye bread**

> **Wheat bread**

> **High-fiber cereals** (frequently check the labels as commercial-brand formulas often change, including more sugar)

> **All Bran®**

> **Bran Buds®**

> **Cracklin' Bran®**

> **Fiber One®**

> **Grapenuts®**

> **Kashi Go Lean®**

> **Oatmeal**

> **Puffed Wheat®**

> **Rolled Oats**

> **Vegetables**

> **Beans**

> **Broccoli**

> **Brussels sprouts**

> **Carrots**

> **Cauliflower**

> **Corn**

> **Greens** (kale, collards, swiss chard, turnip greens)

> **Lentils**

> **Lima beans**

> **Nuts**

> **Peas**

> **Peanuts**

> **Pumpkin seeds**

> **Soybeans**

> **Spinach**

Summary of Orders

> **Eat a small meal every three to four hours** (except while sleeping, of course)

> **Consume a small quantity of quality, low-GI carbs at every meal**

> **Reduce or eliminate high-GI carbs**

> **Include high-fiber foods at several of your small feedings daily**

> **Begin to feel significantly better throughout the day**

BRIEFING #2
Nutrient Purpose: Protein

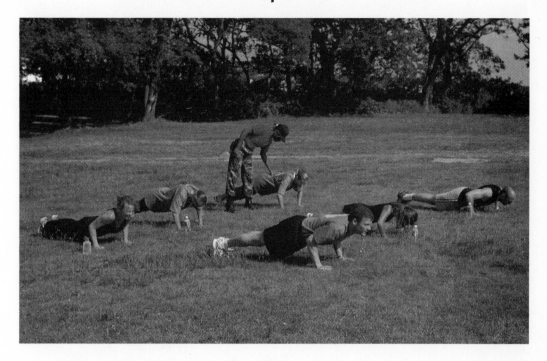

WHEN YOU SHOVELED that tasty chicken breast or a few egg whites into your mouth at chow time, your small intestines released digestive enzymes to break the protein down into its fundamental amino acids. The aminos hitched a ride through your bloodstream to your liver where they were recombined into the proper mixture for building new tissues, bones, muscles, enzymes, hormones, genes, and brain cells. With the proper amount of protein in your diet to meet your training demands, you will properly supply your efforts to gain strength and build shape-giving muscle.

Protein provides your body's building blocks for muscle and other tissues. Although your body can manufacture eleven of the amino acids required to make protein, there are nine that it cannot make and must get from food. Your body has to work hard to digest protein, and that hard work can speed your metabolism by up to 30% for several hours after you finish eating. So, if you included a reasonable amount of protein in your lunch, your body's energy-burning furnace stays active, and you remain more mentally alert and focused through the afternoon than if you focused only on carbs.

When you train, you lose a substantial amount of protein through sweat and loss of red blood cells. Consuming quality protein along with a balanced carbohydrate intake will ensure that you always have enough building materials to produce more muscle and repair all other tissues and that you have the energy to use those building materials efficiently.

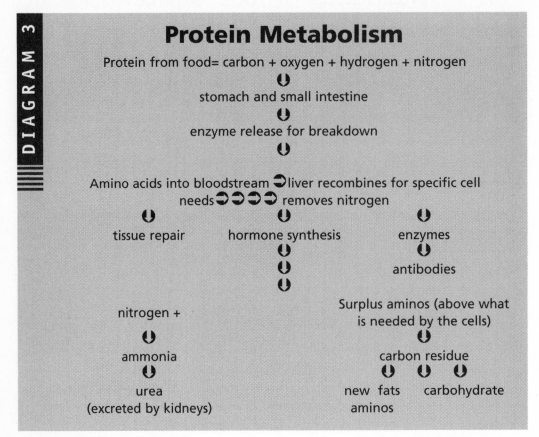

Sources of Protein

Your sources of protein may be either animal or plant-based, but if your objectives include superior physique and performance, you will get a solid amount of your protein from animal sources: whey (a milk protein), egg whites, fish, lean poultry, and occasionally lean meats. You will balance them with plant-source protein for both meal variety and added nutrients.

The two highest-quality sources of protein for use in your body are egg albumin, found in egg whites, and lactalbumin, a milk protein ideally consumed in the form of a whey protein concentrate. These two sources can provide a nearly perfect mix of the amino acids you require in a form that your body readily uses to build muscle and repair tissues. Next in line are fish, poultry, and lean meats. Since you want to avoid the saturated fat that usually comes with your meat supply, you will advance toward chicken and turkey (remove the skin) and fish and shellfish. When you look to the vegetable group for additional protein sources, you should include soybeans and other soy products. Soy provides eight of the nine essential aminos in adequate amounts (you can get a sufficient supply of the remaining amino acids by including brown rice and other grains throughout the day). Other plant foods fill out the bottom of the list of desirable protein sources because individually they don't provide optimal quantities of the essential aminos, but many of them can provide valuable sources of fiber. Keep your balance, Recruit, get your protein from a variety of sources every day, relying primarily on animal sources with a few servings of plant-based protein to keep your diet interesting.

"But I've ignored the kind of teeth that are in my mouth and decided to be a vegetarian!" you whine.

At ease, Recruit! Hopefully, even if you've rejected meat and fish, you've retained the good sense to still eat egg whites and are willing to invest in a quality protein supplement containing whey protein hydrolysates (predigested milk protein). Keeping those options will ensure that you consume quality protein even if you don't eat meat.

If you've made the choice to become a vegan (consuming no products connected with animals in any way), then focus on the health benefits of your training—trying not to die too early—because you're sacrificing your physique and performance potential. Even the health benefits of vegan protein sources are inferior to those provided by whey protein alone. Soy protein has become a headline sweetheart praised for cardiac protection, cholesterol lowering, and cancer prevention. But some of the components of soy (isoflavones) are now suspected to actually increase the risk of cancer in women, and another main ingredient (genistein) significantly drops the testosterone concentration in male rats (the jury's still out on the levels for humans). On the other hand, whey protein has been known for its health benefits since about 400 B.C., when Hippocrates pointed them out. Whey contains all of the essential amino acids, has been shown to prevent the formation of cancer tumors and reduce the progress of existing tumors in both rats and humans, improves immune function, helps fight infection, and lowers bad cholesterol. Whey protein provides the same health benefits as soy and outperforms it with none of the risks. The quality of plant protein for rebuilding muscle and other tissues is simply inferior to the protein found in whey and eggs.

Vegetarians must combine plant-based proteins with grains to get the proper quantities of all the amino acids. However, it's not true that you need to combine them all in the same meal. You probably need to get complete proteins within the same day, but not necessarily at the same sitting.

Your bigger concern, if you don't eat any animal products, is how much plant food you have to devour daily to get all the protein and other nutrients you need. For the 14 grams of protein you get in four egg whites, you have to consume 2 cups of lentils. For the 18 grams of protein that you'd get in a single scoop of a good whey protein powder mixed with juice or water, you can eat 2/3 of a cup of soybeans. Great. But, depending on your body weight and training goals, you may need up to 100 grams of protein today! Not too tough with some scrambled egg whites, a tuna sandwich, a skinless chicken breast, and a scoop or two of a whey protein supplement. More challenging with a cup of split peas, a cup of soybeans, a cup and a half of lima beans, a cup of lentils, and two cups of soy milk. After all that, you'd still have to pile on more food because you haven't yet eaten the carbs you need, and even then you may still run low on zinc, iron, calcium, and vitamin B-12. If you're a strict vegetarian, you'd better be thorough—and hungry!

High-Protein Fads

What about getting more than enough protein? Unless you've been asleep under a rock, you've probably heard the diet scams telling you that protein is the way to go—almost all protein, all the time. If you're old enough to remember the crazy weight-loss ideas of the 70's, including the high-protein and liquid-protein diets, perhaps you also remember the accounts of folks who suffered electrolyte imbalances, serious medical problems, and even death from following this quackery. Well, as a negative example of how history repeats itself, this enemy is back on the battlefield.

If you've stumbled into cookie-cutter recommendations for your nutrient intake (i.e., the same percentages of everything for everyone), or are following the new rogue food pyramid sponsored by the low-carb gurus, you're pretending you can improve your physique with complicated food combinations or by identifying evil nutrients. In fact, you've likely just been on a very low-calorie diet of 800 to 1,200 calories—no magic, just starvation. Worse, if you enlisted in one of the low-carb-diet-with-a-name cults, you've pretended that dizziness, nausea, fatigue, bad breath, and losing water weight and lean muscle instead of body fat are positive things. Hopefully by now you've relocated your brain's "On" button and returned to good judgment!

If you consume very few carbs for fuel and substitute more protein than your body needs for rebuilding, some of the excess protein can be converted to glucose for fuel. So you're thinking, "if protein can be used to make both building blocks and energy, maybe the quacks are right and protein really *is* all I need to eat." Negative!

Here's the part those financially successful wizards don't tell you. Carbs and fats are made of carbon, hydrogen, and oxygen, just like protein. But protein also contains nitrogen. Your body now has an extra element to dispense if it has to convert protein to glucose or fat for energy, so it converts the nitrogen to ammonia. Ammonia is highly toxic so your body converts that to urea and stores it in your kidneys until you urinate to get rid of it. Aside from getting rid of your normal supply of bodily waste, your kidneys then have to work extra hard if your body has to make energy from protein and consequently produces excess urea.

If there's too much protein, and especially if you've reduced or eliminated your other nutrients on a quack diet:

1) **You won't have enough energy to train hard, so you can't take advantage of the faster metabolism that would normally come from improving your physique.**

2) **Your body would rather use the little energy it can muster to stay alive than use it up building new tissue (including muscle), so you will neither maintain nor build lean muscle even with plenty of building blocks.**

3) **You can strain your kidneys, poison your blood, and become susceptible to cancers and other kidney diseases, especially if you have any compromised kidney functioning as is estimated for one in four Americans.**

4) **Recent studies confirm that people on high-protein, carb-restricted diets lose weight at the same rate or just slightly faster than those on other diets—for up to six months. But after a year, they lose no more weight than subjects on other restricted-calorie diets; they do not have lower levels of bad cholesterol (in fact, in some cases, it's higher); and when they can no longer sustain the ridiculous regimen , they gain just as much of the weight back as those on every other fad diet.**

If you start any day's training session without enough glycogen loaded in your muscles (because your new fad diet doesn't let you eat enough carbs), your body will take some of the energy it needs from its protein supply. Since the most accessible protein is now part of the very muscles you need to use when training, you'll actually burn some of that muscle tissue, along with the protein you recently consumed, for fuel. Think! If your body has to switch from running on carbs to running on protein, it cannibalizes the lean muscle you're building in order to keep your vital organs functioning. Does that seem like a good idea to you?

Common sense must prevail. You know that your car needs gas to run and antifreeze to maintain proper operating temperature, so you wouldn't listen to a mechanic who told you to dump antifreeze in the gas tank because the car can learn to run on it. Even if the engine could run for a while on the antifreeze instead of the proper fuel, the vehicle won't perform well and will eventually stop in the middle of the road. Your body is designed to use specific nutrients for specific purposes, and protein's purpose is tissue building. How much muscle you build will always depend on how much, and how hard you train. Substituting protein for carbs leads to inferior muscular performance, lower energy levels, and too much toxic waste. So quit listening to diet quacks. Think!

Direct Order #4:

You will consume a small amount of quality protein in each of your small daily feedings.

Listed below are some better-quality, low-fat, bio-available protein sources you should **ADVANCE TOWARD** and some less preferable, higher-fat protein sources from which you should **RETREAT**. You will inspect your cabinets, pantry, refrigerator, and restaurant menus and make the necessary adjustments:

RETREAT FROM

> **High-fat sources** (they have plenty of protein, but you can get that without the extra lard)

>> **Beef** (even lean)

>> **Pork** (even lean)

>> **Bacon**

>> **Butter**

ADVANCE TOWARD

> **Egg whites**

> **Whey protein concentrate** (see Reference Section for specific product examples)

> **Fish** (especially cold water varieties)**:**

>> **Tuna packed in water** (but choose reputable brands and avoid high mercury levels)

>> **Flounder**

>> **Orange roughy**

>> **Salmon**

>> **Trout**

> **Shellfish**

    > **Clams**

    > **Crabs**

    > **Mussels**

    > **Lobster**

    > **Shrimp**

> **Lean poultry** (skin removed)

    > **Chicken**

    > **Game birds** (such as quail and pheasant)

    > **Ostrich**

    > **Turkey**

> **Lean game**

    > **Buffalo**

    > **Kangaroo**

    > **Ostrich**

    > **Rabbit**

    > **Venison**

> **Beans and legumes**

    > **Black-eye peas**

    > **Black beans**

    > **Dried whole peas**

    > **Kidney beans**

    > **Lentils**

    > **Lima beans**

    > **Navy beans**

    > **Split peas**

    > **Soybeans**

    > **Wheat germ**

> **Tofu and soybean products**

Summary of Orders

> Consume small amounts of protein in each of your daily feedings

> Get the majority of your protein from high-quality animal-based sources, emphasizing whey protein, egg protein, fish, and poultry

> Add plant sources for balance

> Focus on the solid physique that results from being able to train effectively on a balanced diet

BRIEFING #3
Nutrient Purpose: Fats

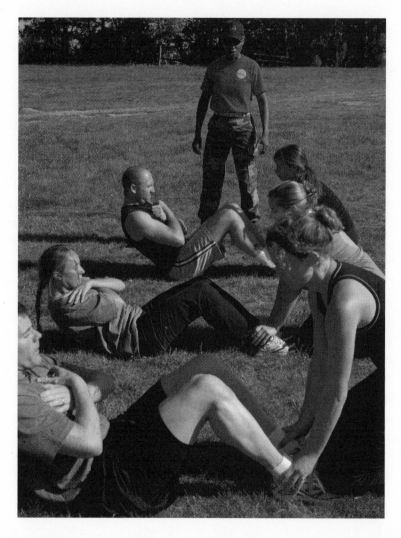

SHORT ANSWERS FIRST: Yes, you need some fat in your diet. Yes, too much fat will make you fatter, but probably not for the reasons you think. No, the majority of the "fat-free" and "low-fat" foods on the market are still not particularly good for you.

Fats are a secondary source of energy for your body. When you had that cream cheese on your bagel this morning, your small intestines released lipase and bile to break it down to free fatty acids, glycerol, cholesterol, and phospholipids all of which made their way to your intestinal wall cells. Those components were then recombined for transport through your bloodstream to your muscles for energy, to storage as body fat, or to your liver for further processing, depending on what your body needed and just how much of it you ate. If you were already well fed on a balanced diet, most of the fat went to storage. If you were not well fed, as on nearly any fad diet, the fatty acids were shipped to your muscles to be used for energy. The fat also helped you metabolize the fat soluble vitamins (A, D, E, and K), provided shock absorption for your internal organs, and, for females, likely helped regulate the menstrual cycle.

"Hey, then that crazy fad diet still doesn't seem so bad. You just said that my body can ship the fat to my muscles and I use fat for energy. I get to eat the fatty foods I like, and I can still use them to fuel my training! Why can't I eat more fat and less brown rice?"

Good questions. It's true that fat provides energy, but your body can *make* most fats from any other nutrient it finds in surplus. You don't need to consume much fat because you're making it daily! Any excess fuel you consume gets shipped off to fat storage; your body still prefers to burn carbs for its energy because the conversion is much more efficient than trying to extract the fuel from fat.

Pay attention here. A calorie is a measure of energy potential, nothing more. Fats contain about 9 calories per gram and carbs contain about 4 calories per gram. So fats hold more than twice as much energy as carbs which makes them seem like a good choice for fuel. But here's the catch: Your body converts fat into ATP, the fuel for action (review Briefing #1), at roughly half the rate at which it extracts the same energy from carbs. Think about it. If you had to wait twice as long in one line at the gas station as in another, wouldn't you choose the line that gets you the gas faster? So would your body. In most individuals, it takes twice as long to get the fuel from fats, so it's more efficient for your body to get it from carbs.

Most people who are working to lose that gut or the love handles need to engage in activities that will allow the most efficient burning of fats for fuel. That activity will be low-intensity (70 to 80% of your estimated maximum heart rate), longer-lasting aerobic exercise (more than 30 minutes). Performing this type of exercise will help most people burn significantly more stored fat than carbohydrate for energy. If you are working to lose fat, then, you would not want to consume excessive amounts of dietary fat because you're just boosting the supply you're trying to reduce.

The exception here is for highly trained endurance athletes because serious, high-level training increases the body's ability to use fat efficiently. Essentially, if your activity level gets high enough, your body will learn to convert everything available into useable fuel to meet the activity demand. These athletes' performance is typically enhanced with increased consumption of dietary fat because the body can simply store more fat than it can carbohydrates (remember, it converts excess carbs into fat for storage). It can then tap those fat stores for the energy required to continue performing at high intensities for long periods of time. Don't get excited, Recruit. The activity level we're talking about for you to make that kind of conversion is 90 minutes or more of *continuous* aerobic exercise, daily. And with high consumption of saturated fats linked to increases in cholesterol levels, cardiovascular disease, heart attacks and death, you are advised to keep your fat intake relatively low unless you're training at an elite level for endurance activities and are sure you have no family history of heart problems or high cholesterol.

"But if I already have too much body fat, doesn't restricting carbs make my body burn the fat? Who cares if it converts more slowly on my fad diet, at least it'll burn, right?"

Listen up, Recruit. When you restrict the preferred energy source, your body doesn't just open the fat supplies and start burning. It burns all the stored carbohydrate it can find first (muscle and liver glycogen, see Briefing #1) and you also lose water because every gram of that carbohydrate is attached to 2.5 grams of water. Then your body tries to suck some energy from the protein in your tissues (especially muscles) and the food you eat. You might reduce some body fat, but you don't have enough energy to build anything impressive of the flabby carcass that's left. Increasing your fat intake without maintaining your body's carb stores, as encouraged on many low-carb plans, will hurt your training performance; unless you're already a hardcore, elite-level endurance athlete, you won't have the physical energy to keep working for long.

There are only two essential fats, ones that your body can't manufacture—linoleic acid and alpha-linolenic acid. They are the only two fats you must eat. Of course, we all know those aren't the only fats you're going to eat. Even those who don't eat animal products will get a small amount of fat from plant foods, so you will focus on keeping your fat intake low while getting the essential fats you require.

Direct Order #5:

Consume only very small amounts of fat daily and focus on foods that provide linoleic acid and alpha-linolenic acid, the only essential fats.

DIAGRAM 4

Structure of Fats

C: Carbon
H: Hydrogen
O: Oxygen
+ : single bond – a C atom is attached to as many H atoms as possible in each direction
++ : double bond – two C atoms share two pairs of electrons and are joined directly together on one side (no H in that spot)

Sample Saturated Fat - Butyric acid (in butter)

```
        H    H    H    O
        +    +    +    ++
    H + C +  C +  C +  C
        +    +    +    +
        H    H    H    O+H
```

Sample Monunsaturated Fat – Oleic acid (olive oil)

```
O    H   H   H   H   H   H   H            H   H   H   H   H   H   H   H
++   +   +   +   +   +   +   +            +   +   +   +   +   +   +   +
C +  C + C + C + C + C + C + C +C++ C +   C + C + C + C + C + C + C + H
+    +   +   +   +   +   +   +   +        +   +   +   +   +   +   +   +
O+H  H   H   H   H   H   H   H   H        H   H   H   H   H   H   H   H
```

Sources of Fats

As with all of your nutrients, there are preferred sources of your dietary fat and sources you should avoid. You've already heard a few things in the press and probably from your doctor about saturated and unsaturated fats. Those terms simply refer to the type of fatty acid that makes up the fat you eat. To review, fat contains carbon, oxygen, and hydrogen like all the other nutrients. This time, the key player is the hydrogen. Load a fatty acid up with all the hydrogen it can hold and it is saturated and solid at room temperature (think: butter and other animal fats). Find a fatty acid that has some open slots free for hydrogen and it's unsaturated and liquid at room temperature (think: vegetable oils). If the unsaturated fat has only one slot open, it's a monounsaturated fat (these are your best bet, as you'll see later); if it has a few slots open, it's a polyunsaturated fat. As explained above, the fat in your diet is broken down into fatty acids, glycerol, cholesterol and phospholipids. The liver then adds some protein to form various lipoproteins.

The type of lipoproteins formed depends on how much of each fat component is present, and you know them better by their initials: "LDL" and "HDL." Although we commonly call these two compounds "cholesterol," you can see now that cholesterol is only one of their components. The summary: Low-density lipoprotein (LDL) carries more cholesterol and is the bad guy and high-density lipoprotein (HDL) carries more protein and is a better critter. Here's the scoop.

LDL travels through the bloodstream gathering even more cholesterol from your liver and dropping it off in other cells in your body; this cholesterol can then be absorbed into your artery walls. All those cholesterol deliveries can cause a traffic jam in your blood vessels—like freight being trucked on the same route you take to work. Eventually your blood, the real commuter, can't make it through anymore. If the jammed thruway happens to be a highway to your heart, the traffic jam is coronary heart disease and you're standing by for a heart attack!

HDL also travels with a cholesterol load, but it moves in the opposite direction bringing that cholesterol back from your body's cells to your liver to be further broken down or redirected. This is the traffic cop you'd like to have helping out on your commute—redirect the wide loads, keep thruways flowing, send slow moving vehicles back to the garage. With higher HDL levels, you will help avoid many coronary issues and clogged artery problems.

Saturated fat, weighed down with its hydrogen load, helps raise your LDL levels, drags artery-clogging trash along with it, and thereby increases your risk of heart disease, heart attack, and stroke. Unsaturated fats, especially monounsaturated, take a much more active part in your biological functions, including key roles in keeping your brain, ears, eyes, adrenal glands, and sex organs healthy. Recruits who consume more monounsaturated fats and eliminate the saturated fats will help raise their HDL levels and lower their LDL. Now, if you've been reading the claims of some of the fad diet gurus, you know that they cite research showing that the higher fat intake they recommend does NOT lead to coronary problems. You need to read a little closer...

Although short-term studies show positive training effects and a lack of increased cardiac risk with higher fat intake, these tests have been done on highly trained, very active individuals who showed no signs or family history of obesity. And the studies done on overweight subjects actually show an increase in the levels of LDL cholesterol with low-carb, high-protein, high-fat diets. Obviously, there is no surprise in the fact that if you decide to put economy fuel instead of premium in your high-performance sports car one afternoon, you'll still probably blow everybody else off the freeway. But low-grade fuel doesn't speed up the old family sedan at all. Smarten up, lower your fat intake—especially saturated fats—and burn the better fuel.

One more thing, your processed foods often contain fats that started out on the better-for-you unsaturated list, but the manufacturers ruin them by adding hydrogen to the open slots. I'm talking about the partially hydrogenated oils you see listed on your food labels. Pay attention now, this is a sneaky one.

You read a label and see that the product contains soybean oil.

"Excellent," you think. "That's on the 'Advance Toward' list at the end of this section."

Stop. What are those two words that come right before it on the label? "Partially hydrogenated?" Then put it down. Those pesky food packagers take an otherwise good for you, monounsaturated vegetable oil and add more hydrogen to the empty slots on the fat's chain making the fat more saturated. Apparently, doing this helps to increase the product's shelf life and, of course, makes it tastier. But that's not so good for you. You may think you're doing well because you're getting a healthy vegetable oil, but if it's partially hydrogenated it's been turned into one of the bad guys. Avoid it.

Direct Order #6:

Stay alert on your post—keep your saturated fats to an absolute minimum, get your essential fats, and keep the rest of your fat intake monounsaturated.

Listed below are the better-quality, unsaturated fat sources you should **ADVANCE** toward and the less preferable saturated fats from which you should **RETREAT**. Adjust!

RETREAT FROM

> **Bacon**

> **Bologna**

> **Butter** (note: a small amount is still a better choice than the harmful trans-fats in margarine)

> **Cheddar cheese**

> **Cream cheese** (choose fat-free varieties)

> **Fake fats** (as in some diet foods—the worst ones can strip your body of fat-soluble vitamins, the best maintain your taste for fats and make limiting the real ones even harder)

> **Pork roast**

> **Pork sausage**

> **T-bone steak**

> **Tropical fats and oils**

>> **Palm**

>> **Palm kernel**

>> **Coconut**

> **Egg yolks**

> **Frankfurters**

ADVANCE TOWARD

> **Cottage cheese** (1% fat)

> **Fish and shellfish**

>> **Cod**

>> **Crab**

>> **Flounder**

>> **Halibut**

>> **Herrings**

>> **Mussels**

>> **Salmon**

>> **Sardines**

>> **Scallops**

>> **Shrimp**

>> **Sole**

>> **Tuna**

> **Lean/low-cholesterol meats**

>> **Buffalo steak**

>> **Chicken breast**

>> **Lamb**

>> **Turkey breast**

>> **Veal**

> **Rice bran**

> **Ricotta cheese**

> Unsaturated oils

  > Almond

  > Canola

  > Corn

  > Flaxseed

  > Safflower

  > Sesame

  > Sunflower

  > Soybean

  > Virgin olive

  > Walnut

> Foods rich in essential fats

  > Salmon

  > Sardines

  > Mackerel

  > Soybeans

  > Walnuts

  > Pumpkin seeds

  > Canola oil

Summary of Orders

> You will consume small amounts of fat daily.

> You will include foods that provide linoleic acid and alpha-linolenic acid, the only essential fats.

> You will work to reduce, preferably eliminate, saturated fats and consume more monounsaturated fats.

BRIEFING #4
Staying Hydrated

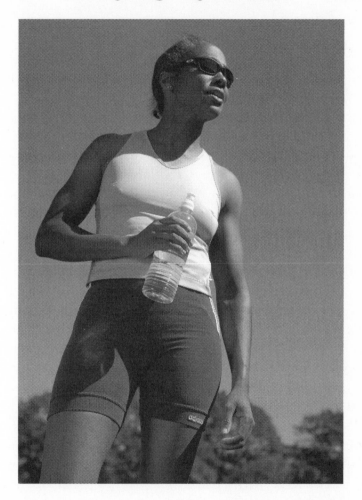

RECRUIT, THIS REALLY SHOULD BE A NO-BRAINER: Drink your water. It's a simple habit, easy to do, inexpensive. So why do most Recruits walk around almost dangerously dehydrated most of the time? No excuse!

You've heard since high school biology that your body is more than ¾ water. You've probably had a hard time picturing it, but it's true. Take a look at the list of the percentage of water that makes up some vital organs.

Percentage of major body parts that is composed of water

> Bones   25%

> Liver   96%

> Kidneys   83%

> Muscles   75%

> Brain   75%

> Blood   82%

> Lungs   86%

> Heart   75%

Now think of other common water-filled items and what happens if the fluid isn't regularly refilled. Do you have an aquarium? How quickly will the fish be swimming upside down if you don't keep adding more water? Got pets? Hopefully, you fill their bowls daily with fresh water or they'll collapse within the week. Soak the sponge you use in the kitchen. Leave it on the shelf and it'll be dry as a bone in a day or so. And none of those things does what you do in a day.

The basic requirement is eight to ten 8-ounce glasses of water daily just to keep you functioning normally. That's a bare minimum requirement, and most recruits I meet don't even drink that much. When you engage in light activity in 70–degree weather at about 70% humidity, you lose those eight glasses of water in less than an hour. You operate at a water deficit for the rest of the day if you don't drink more. If you train any harder or in any warmer weather, you will lose even more water— water that has to be replaced—throughout your activity period. Still skeptical?

Check your scale. Your body won't burn more than about 2 pounds of body fat a week regardless of what diet you're following. In most cases, any more rapid weight loss simply means that you're losing water and possibly muscle if your body is struggling to find an energy source (i.e., if you're eating too few calories or insufficient carbs). Realistic fat loss only adds up to about ¼ pound a day. So just weigh yourself before and immediately after your next training session. If you're training as hard as you should be, you're probably at least 2 to 4 pounds lighter after training. Now think hard, Recruit. There are 16 ounces in a pound and you're at least 32 ounces lighter. No more than about 4 ounces of that could be fat. You have to account for a minimum of 28 ounces of weight lost while training. Guess what, it's water. And that's 3½ glasses you need to drink right there.

Need more ways to measure whether you're properly hydrated? You should have to urinate several times every day (but if it keeps you up at night, you may need to adjust your timing or get a med check to rule out any more serious problems.) When you are well hydrated, your urine should be thin and clear. If it's concentrated, dark, or brightly colored; if you only have to go once or twice a day; or if you go infrequently but the volume is still small—you need to drink more.

Pay attention to your energy level. If you're getting enough sleep and you've corrected your feeding schedule, but you still feel tired or unfocused during the day, chances are you need more water. Back in Marine Corps officer training when as young candidates we spent our days running around in the Virginia heat—trying to execute drill commands, sneaking through the woods practicing combat tactics, and cleaning everything from rifles to toilets—we sometimes had trouble staying awake through classroom instruction even after the 8 hours of sleep clearly provided on our training schedule. The remedy enforced, as a head bounced precariously toward a desktop, usually involved drinking a full canteen of water. And it worked. Staying hydrated should help you stay alert.

So what's the big deal? What does water actually do for you? For one thing, water provides the environment in which all other nutrients function. Here are a few more key functions of water you should think about.

> **It controls your electrolyte balance to maintain cell functioning.**

> **It provides the building material for cell protoplasm which is the essence of your entire physical self.**

> **It transports every compound in your body—nutrients in and waste out.**

> **It helps all your senses function, transmitting hearing waves, reflecting light in your inner eye, and dissolving foods and odors for taste and smell.**

> **It regulates acid levels in your body.**

> **It regulates your body temperature so you can move around without passing out even when the air temperature, humidity, or excess clothing raises your core body temperature.**

Keeping all systems working well takes more water than most people drink. Start with the basic requirement of 64 ounces (two quarts) every day. When you train moderately on any given day, drink another quart. When you train hard, when the temperature climbs above 70 degrees Fahrenheit, or if the humidity is higher than 70%, drink at least another quart.

Direct Order #7:

You will drink at least 16 glasses of water (a gallon) on training days and at least 8 glasses on non-training days.

Recruits always want to know whether all of the fluid replacement has to come from water. Can you count juice, water-loaded fruits and vegetables, and other beverages? With the exception of diuretics like caffeine and alcohol—substances that suck moisture out of the body by causing you to urinate more without replacing that water—all fluids can count toward your hydration efforts. But one problem is that the solids in some of these tasty fluid sources interfere with your body's ability to absorb the water quickly. Sugars and the laundry list of ingredients in your favorite beverage all have to first get out of your stomach to your intestines where the water gets absorbed and shipped out to work in other organs. You also have to account for additional calories you may take in with every sip of some of these beverages.

Now comes the slightly self-righteous aerobics refugee from the rear of the squad, "I only drink caffeine-free, sugar-free, diet soda or sparkling water. What's wrong with that?" Not much. Except that the phosphoric acid found in many sodas may lead to kidney stones and the bubbles in your sparkling water or clear sodas can make you make you feel so full that you don't want to drink as much fluid as you would if the water were flat. Look, Recruit, you can get some water from almost everything. It's the most abundant substance on earth. Your orders are to get as much as your body needs to keep all systems functioning well. So drink your juices and eat your fruits, but include at least two quarts of water every day to make sure you're well hydrated!

"Okay, but can't I get too much water? I saw in a newspaper article where a marathon runner died from it."

In a nutshell: Hyponatraemia is a rare condition that can occur when the body's supply of sodium and other electrolytes become too diluted with excess water. It is relatively common among hospital patients because they are often given drugs that affect many aspects of their bodies' chemical balance while trying to make them well. The condition has been seen increasingly in extreme endurance event athletes who have typically drunk copious quantities of water without consuming much food, which would contain enough sodium to keep everything balanced. Having been told that their exertion levels require them to be extremely well hydrated, these athletes often continue to drink only water and are often too worried about intestinal upset or getting slowed down on the road to eat snacks during their event. While running up to 100 miles or trekking through the wilderness for a few days, they lose moisture and sodium through sweat, drink more and more water, and begin to experience intracranial pressure when their brain cells start to swell as fluid shifts from outside the cells to the inside. Soon, they experience massive headaches, nausea, vomiting, confusion, seizures, and possibly unconsciousness and death. That's very bad.

Now, be serious about your own situation. Reaching the point where you've lost most of the salt in your body is very rare. Presumably, you are not currently hospitalized; and even if you are, your doctors and nurses will work to correct your sodium levels. Under normal circumstances, nearly everything you will choose to eat in our modern society (and certainly everything you're ordered to include on this mission) should provide enough electrolytes to keep you balanced. If your goals include extreme endurance activities—aerobic activity lasting more than an hour continuously or work in very hot environments—just include proper nutrition along with your frequent water breaks, include a diluted sports drink at every other break, and you should be fine.

Summary of Orders

> Drink at least 16 glasses of water (a gallon) on training days and at least 8 glasses on non-training days.

> Avoid sugared beverages and carbonated sodas.

> If you drink sparkling water or clear sodas, make sure you drink enough to meet your hydration requirements and, preferably, include several glasses of pure, water.

BRIEFING #5:

Nutrient Balance: How Much Do You Need?

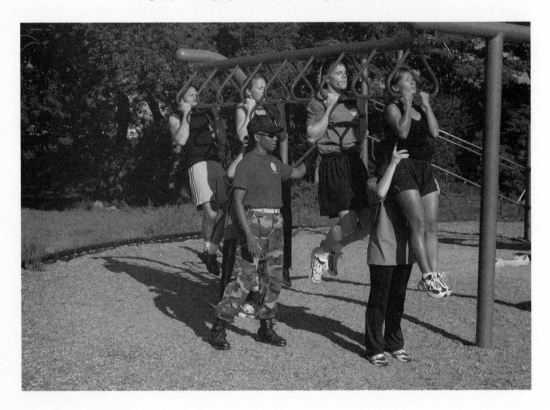

"HOW MUCH FOOD SHOULD I BE EATING, how much of each nutrient do I need, and why am I just getting this detail now?" you boldly inquire.

I'll answer that last question first. For starters, Recruit, you had enough to worry about just trying to correct your eating schedule and making sure you consume quality fuel. In many cases, increasing the frequency of your meals without making a single adjustment to your total caloric intake can help you start to reduce your body fat and give you more energy. That was the first step. Now that you're thinking clearly about what the fuel does and why you eat, you will learn how to calculate how much of it you need to reach your objectives.

You will arrive at your nutrient requirements by:

1) determining your estimated energy expenditure (how many calories your body tries to burn during your normal daily activities).

2) determining your target daily Caloric intake to start operating efficiently and working toward your objectives.

3) calculating your target protein intake to build quality muscle and maintain your lean mass without overloading your system with by-product waste.

4) calculating your target fat intake so you keep all systems operating smoothly and minimize storage.

5) calculating your target carb intake, the high-octane fuel your body wants—and needs—to run on.

When figuring out how much of each nutrient you need to consume to build your performance machine, the first guidelines we have to discuss are the U.S. Dietary Reference Intakes (DRI).

The development of the DRI was co-sponsored by the Food and Nutrition Board of the U.S. National Academies and Health Canada. They are intended to replace the Recommended Dietary Allowance (RDA) by accounting for new nutrient information, the need to help reduce chronic disease in the U.S. and Canadian populations, and the need to identify how much is too much for any given nutrient. Over the previous five decades the RDA guidelines typically recommended too many calories for most people's activity levels (2,200 calories a day for adult women and 2,900 calories a day for men), miniscule amounts of protein (8 to 9% of total caloric intake), far too much fat (30% of total calories), and high carbs regardless of activity level (about 61%). For years, regular folks assumed this balance was right for all Americans on a daily basis. Meanwhile, we watched ourselves grow fatter by the decade.

The RDA was filled with problems, not the least of which was that people assumed they were guidelines that applied to everyone. Wrong answer. Two primary problems were that the studies on which these recommendations were based for more than 50 years were all done on sedentary individuals, so following the guidance would never have made you anything but just as flabby and weak as the test subjects. In addition, from the beginning, the guidelines were intended only as basic requirements for keeping a representative population alive and generally not sick over a period of time. According to the RDA handbook, "The RDA should not be confused with requirements for a specific individual." Especially if that individual needs to do anything more strenuous than change TV channels!

Now come the improved guidelines. Unfortunately, the new reference still appears to have serious limitations for all but average, sedentary members of the population. The DRI now contains four categories of guidelines:

> **An updated RDA, which is intended to provide the average amount of each nutrient to provide good basic nutrition for 97 to 98% of the healthy people within a particular age range and gender.**

> **The adequate intake recommendations that are to be used for the same purpose as the RDA when an RDA can't be determined.**

> **The estimated average requirement guidelines, which should estimate the appropriate average intake of each nutrient for half of the healthy members of a group within a particular age range and gender.**

> **The tolerable upper intake level guide, which shows the highest amount of each nutrient that will not likely pose a health threat to nearly all of the general population.**

Confusing, eh?

Long story short, these guidelines do not provide much meaningful guidance to anyone other than couch potatoes. In fact, despite the government's presumably strong interest in reversing the current obesity epidemic and excessive burdens to the health care system, none of these guidelines provides information on adequate amounts of any nutrient that might either help sedentary individuals improve their weight, body composition, and health, or help active people properly fuel their training efforts.

The old RDA listed the minimum amount of specific nutrients needed to prevent nutritional deficiencies in population groups; the new DRI shows the minimum amounts necessary to prevent chronic disease along with estimated safe upper limits for daily intake. The new guidelines tell you how little you can consume if you don't want to get sick and how much will make you sick; they still don't tell you how much to eat for optimal benefit.

Your daily requirements are probably different from the DRI for most nutrients, and we will address the basics—how much carbohydrate, fiber, protein, and fat you need to help achieve your objectives. With most of our food currently produced in the presence of polluted soil and air and with the help of staggering amounts of hormones, antibiotics, and other additives, minimum requirements will not help anyone perform or look any better. As you learn to train harder and work more efficiently and as you get leaner and faster and stronger, you must make the time to review your nutritional requirements and check reliable sources about additional nutrients and supplements you may require to perform at your best. You will find more resources to consult regarding supplementation in the Reference section (page 143). For the time being, you need to calculate your basic nutrition requirements.

Now, stay awake, Recruit. We've got to do some math here, but we're going to do it step-by-step so you don't miss anything. Start by breaking out your Recruit Field Journal and a calculator; keep both close by as you crunch the numbers.

Calculating Total Caloric Requirements

When you want to know how much it will cost you to drive to Aunt Millie's for the weekend, you find out how much gas your car's tank holds, how many miles you get to the gallon, and how far you have to go. To estimate your optimal intake for each nutrient and whether you need to eat less, more, or the same to reach your objective, you have to start by learning how much fuel your body is burning—or trying to burn—now. You will estimate how much fuel you're burning by calculating an estimate of your Daily Energy Expenditure Rate.

Your energy expenditure rate represents your estimated Resting Metabolic Rate (RMR) combined with your daily activity expenditure. (RMR is also known as the Basal Energy Expenditure Rate and the Basal Metabolic Rate if you're reading other sources, but we'll stick with RMR here). Your estimated Daily Energy Expenditure Rate represents the amount of energy you'd need just to breathe plus the amount you use doing whatever it is that you do all day.

Your RMR represents the amount of energy your body needs to keep vital systems functioning at rest (breathing, circulation, brain functioning, etc.). Precise calculation of your metabolic rate would require a lab or hospital setting and expensive equipment. Instead, you will estimate your energy requirements using a standard formula, called the Harris-Benedict formula, and standard multipliers to account for your activity level. Record your numbers in the Nutrition Requirements section of your Recruit Field Journal. (You'll notice that the formulas and instructions for calculating your requirements are repeated in your Recruit Field Journal, so you'll be able to review these steps each time you update your information.)

Step One—Estimate Your Daily Energy Expenditure Rate

Use one of the following formulas, depending on your gender, to estimate your RMR. And just in case you've forgotten high school math, Recruit, the stuff in parentheses has to be done first, moving left to right.

FEMALES:

661 + (weight in lbs. x 4.38) + (height in inches x 4.33) – (age in years x 4.7) = _____ (RMR)

MALES:

67 + (weight in lbs. x 6.24) + (height in inches x 12.7) – (age in years x 6.8) = _____ (RMR)

Record your estimated RMR in your Recruit Field Journal.

Now, multiply your estimated RMR by one of the following values to account for your daily activity level. Remember, your multiplier must reflect the actual amount of time you spend performing activities, Recruit. Don't count three days of socializing at the gym if you're only lifting for 15 minutes total each day; that only adds up to one day of training!

Activity Multipliers

> **If you are currently inactive *and* have crash dieted in the past, multiply your RMR by .9**

> **If you are currently inactive but have never crash dieted, multiply your RMR by 1.2**

> **If you are lightly active, exercising 3 days a week for at least an hour, without a physically demanding job or daily activities, multiply your RMR by 1.3**

> **If you are moderately active, exercising 4- to 5 days a week for at least an hour, multiply your RMR by 1.5**

> **If you are very active, exercising for 5- to 6 days each week for at least an hour, multiply your RMR by 1.7**

> **If you are extremely active, exercising daily for more than an hour, training for endurance sports, or engaging in physically demanding, continuous work daily, multiply your resting rate by 1.9**

The result is your estimated Daily Energy Expenditure Rate, the number of calories your body needs to keep you exactly where you are now—at your current weight, performing the activities you normally do.

Record your Daily Energy Expenditure Rate in your Recruit Field Journal.

"What?!" you sputter once again without permission, "But I don't eat nearly that many calories, and I'm still fat!" Or, another popular complaint, "If I start to eat that much I'll get fat!"

At ease, Recruit! Review Briefing #1. Even if you eat less now, if you're overweight it means that at some point you started expending less than you were consuming. Maybe it started with larger meals. Maybe it was continuing to eat like the team captain long after the last game ended. Maybe it was binge eating out of boredom, frustration, anger, loneliness, or some combination. No matter how it started, eating more than you burned helped you construct that flabby gut. Your metabolism learns slowly to store excess fat without burning it. Now it tries to maintain its current state—whatever that may be—and doesn't react well to sharp, sudden changes.

If you're thin but flabby, you may still be overfat and need to correct your intake.

If you're eating significantly less than what's required for a creature your size, your metabolism has likely slowed with the panic of starvation. If you've always stayed undernourished, your body never had a chance to operate properly. Even if you haven't supplied the necessary calories from food, your body has maintained its pudgy mass by burning the glycogen from your muscles, storing more body fat for fuel reserves, and keeping your energy level low so you can't perform much activity.

So now you have to determine the number of calories that will best fuel your training efforts. If you do not need to change your body weight, you will consume the same number of calories you just calculated as your Daily Energy Expenditure Rate to maintain balance. If you need to change your body weight by more than about 5 pounds, you will adjust your caloric intake to achieve those goals. You will repeat these nutrient requirement calculations every time your body weight changes by 10 pounds (sooner if you get stuck on a plateau for more than 2 weeks).

Calorie Count

> **If you do not need to change your body weight, your total calories should equal your calculated Daily Energy Expenditure Rate.**

> **If you need to lose weight, reduce your Daily Energy Expenditure Rate by 30%, but by no more than 500 calories.**

> **If you need to gain weight, increase your Daily Energy Expenditure Rate by 30%, but by no more than 500 calories.**

EXAMPLE: A male who needs to lose 20 pounds has estimated his Daily Energy Expenditure Rate at 2,800 calories per day. He calculates that a 30% caloric reduction would have him drop 840 calories daily, so he chooses the alternative maximum of 500 calories instead, and will recalculate his needs when he's dropped 10 pounds

Daily Energy Expenditure Rate of 2,800 calories x .30 = 840 fewer calories, but that's too much

500 calories = maximum acceptable reduction

2,800—500 = 2,300 target calories daily to start his weight loss

Again, as your body composition changes and you begin to make desirable weight changes on your mission, you will recalculate your nutrition requirements. You'll become very familiar with the equations, but here's another example to get you started.

Private Jefferson is a 40-year-old, 5'4", 165 pound woman who wants to reduce her body weight to fall within reasonable guidelines. She has just begun *Boot Camp Abs* training for one hour, 3 days a week. She works at a desk job, runs the usual errands after most days' work, does housecleaning and yard work on the weekends, and takes an occasional ski trip.

Using the formula for women:

661 + (165 lbs. x 4.38) + (64 inches x 4.33) − (40 years x 4.7) = 1,473 calories (estimated RMR)

She multiplies her estimated RMR by 1.3 to represent her new "lightly active" activity level:

1,473 x 1.3 = 1,915 calories Daily Energy Expenditure Rate

She subtracts 30% to estimate the number of calories she must eliminate to help her reduce body fat while sufficiently fueling her training activities:

1,915 x .30 = 574

Thirty percent is slightly high for her, so she accepts the 500 calorie maximum reduction and subtracts that from her energy expenditure rate to get her new daily target.

1,915—500 = 1,415 target daily caloric intake

Now turn back to your Recruit Field Journal nutrition worksheets, plug in your own numbers, and record your target daily caloric intake.

Once we know how many total calories you need daily, we have to find the proper balance so you can meet your goals. Because most recruits' goals involve basic conditioning rather than elite-level sport performance, we'll stick to fundamental requirements. If your goals include more substantial muscle mass or elite-level performance, your nutrient balance requirements may be different. You will refer to the Reference section for additional sources to help you with higher-level objectives.

The RDA for protein was .8 gram per kilogram of body weight (enough to keep a hypothetical population of sedentary folks strong enough to change the TV channels), and the DRI recommends using that figure as well. The problem is that your body operates differently when it's challenged through exercise. Your muscles grow because protein supplies the building materials when you train. More importantly, you lose protein through sweat, the death of red blood cells, and your body's own need for more energy when you train. You have to maintain nitrogen balance by getting enough protein in your diet to keep your training and other activities anabolic. "Anabolism" means that your body efficiently makes complex material like muscle from simple substances like food, vitamins, and minerals. If you're out of nitrogen balance, you enter "catabolism" in which your body begins to break down its own tissues, including muscle, trying to get enough fuel to keep you going.

Once you're in training, Recruit, you need more protein than just the stay-alive requirements. On this mission, you are working to improve your strength, endurance, and physique through training that lasts about an hour a day (including your ab work, of course). We're assuming your typical day requires no more than an

124

extra hour of vigorous physical activity. So for your purposes, you will consume 1.4 grams of protein for every kilogram of your body weight, daily. Recruits who engage in other sport activities or vigorous physical labor that brings their total strenuous activity time to more than 3 hours daily must increase that baseline; if you fall into that category, refer to the Reference section (page 143) for further guidance. To achieve your objectives, your requirements are based on averages of the lowest amounts of protein that have been shown to adequately support average level strength and endurance athletes.

With 4 calories in every gram, your protein requirements will likely add up to 20 to 35% of your target daily intake. So let's calculate how much protein you must consume each day.

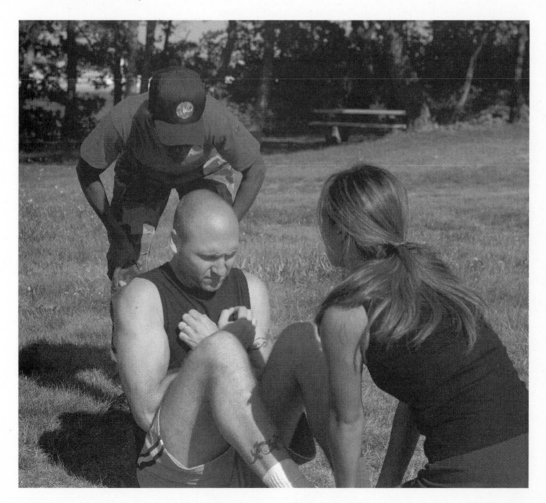

Step Two: Estimating Protein Requirements

First, convert your body weight to kilograms:

(Body weight in lbs.) ÷ 2.2 = _____ kg

Then multiply your body weight in kilograms by 1.4:

(Body weight in kg) x 1.4 = _____ g target protein intake daily

Finally, note how many calories those protein grams will be contributing to your daily intake:

(target protein in grams) x 4 = _____ total calories from protein

EXAMPLE: Private Jefferson converts her body weight of 165 pounds to kilograms and then calculates her protein requirement.

165 ÷ 2.2 = 75 kg

75 x 1.4 grams protein = 105 protein grams daily

105 g protein x 4 = 420 calories from protein

Record your target protein intake in your Recruit Field Journal.

Dietary Fat

Because you require only a small amount of essential fat in your diet, and because your body will make fat from any nutrient it finds in excess, recreational athletes and sedentary people should functional well with less than the 20 to 35% of daily calories from fat as recommended by the DRI and certainly less than the up to 50% that's permitted with some fad diets. Eating fats tends to make you eat more overall because fatty foods are calorically dense. At 9 calories per gram, a small serving of fatty food packs a huge amount of calories. Your body will eventually find that you've consumed more than enough energy, but your mouth and your brain let you keep eating because they don't think you're full after the few small bites you've taken. If that weren't enough, those who are obese (and even those who were obese and have lost the weight) don't appear to use fat efficiently, so they continue to store more of the fat they eat. Convincing patterns shown in thousands of people who have actually succeeded at long-term weight loss indicate that you need to eat fewer fatty foods if you want to keep the weight off. To help you perform at your best, and lose any payload of excess body fat, you must consume no more than 15% of your daily calories from fat and work to reduce or eliminate the saturated fats as much as possible.

Step Three: Estimating Target Fat Intake

First, determine how many calories equals 15% of your Daily Target Caloric Intake:

Target calories x .15 = _____ target fat calories

Target fat calories ÷ 9 calories per gram = _____ g target fat intake daily

EXAMPLE: Private Jefferson has calculated that she requires 1,415 calories daily to start working toward her objective. She determines how much to get from fat as follows:

1,415 x .15 = 212 target fat calories daily

212 ÷ 9 = 23 target grams of fat daily

Record your target fat intake in your Recruit Field Journal.

Now balance it all out with carbohydrates

Once you know how much protein and fat you need to eat, you will get your remaining calories from low-GI carbs. Most recruits will find that their carb requirements add up to approximately 50 to 65% of their total calories, which is important for maintaining proper brain and muscle functioning while fueling your training efforts. You've already calculated the energy supplied from your protein and fat targets. Now you'll subtract those totals from your total target calories; the remainder will come from carbs. Do it step by step.

Step Four: Estimating Target Carb Intake

Add your total fat and protein calories:

Protein calories + fat calories = _____ protein and fat calories

Subtract your fat and protein calories from your Daily Target Caloric Intake:

Daily target caloric intake – protein and fat calories = _____ target carb calories

Then convert your carb calories to grams:

Target carb calories x 4 = _____ g target carb intake in grams

EXAMPLE: Private Jefferson now knows she needs no more than 23 grams of fat for 212 fat calories daily. She also knows she needs 105 grams of protein for 420 calories daily. She subtracts that total from her target caloric intake of 1,415 calories daily, and converts the result to grams to learn how much carbohydrate she will eat:

212 fat calories + 420 protein calories = 632 protein and fat calories

1,415 Daily Target Caloric Intake – 632 protein and fat calories = 783 target carb calories

783 target carb calories ÷ 4 calories per gram = 198 target carb grams daily

Record your carb requirements in your Recruit Field Journal and remember that you need to include 25 to 30 grams of fiber within that daily selection of carbs.

Phew—that was a pack full of numbers! Take a deep breath and rest your brain for a minute, Recruit.

Okay, that's enough.

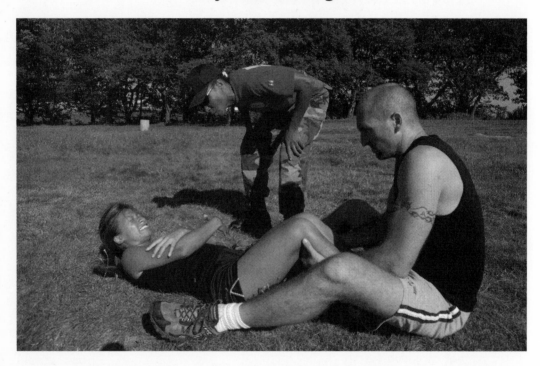

If you live in the U.S. you may be wondering why we bother converting everything into grams when we talk about nutrition. Well, although you probably measure everything at the grocery store and in your kitchen in ounces and pounds, it's all metric in the worlds of nutrition and science. To make the necessary changes in your diet, you must begin to read the labels on the foods you eat carefully, and those labels conform to international standards by showing you your foods' contents in grams and milligrams. Now be smart, Recruit, and learn to read both the Nutrition Facts chart and the ingredients list on every label to see what's really in your food. The

Nutrition Facts chart, now required by U.S. federal law for all food products, provides an overview of the nutrients in your food by total amount as well as by their percentage of a hypothetical daily caloric total.

Straightforward? Simple? Well, if you do your homework it is.

The numbers you're given are per serving, so first you need to determine what the manufacturer calls a serving size. In my experience, unless you're dealing with products that only come in single servings, the designated serving size is often far less than what the average Recruit really eats in one sitting. Don't fool yourself into believing that you're only getting 2 grams of fat from those "low-fat" cookies if the serving size is three cookies and you just popped eight of them into your mouth!

Next, you should focus on the amounts listed for each nutrient rather than the percentage of daily values that appears on the right side of the label.

"But why? Wouldn't it be easier for me to just plug these percentages into my daily targets to stay on track?"

What we have here is the old "sample population" problem. The Daily Values are based on a 2,000 calorie-a-day diet. Now that you've calculated your intake requirements, you know that that may or may not be your optimal target intake. And even if your numbers landed squarely on the 2,000 calorie estimate, the daily values are still the old RDA figures. Using these percentages will get you only 10% protein, a standard 60% carbohydrate, and a whopping 30% fat daily. Your calculations have likely yielded very different targets for your goals. So stick with the grams and keep checking your math.

Finally, knowing the amount of each nutrient still doesn't tell you the quality of the sources in the product. For that, you also need to use the ingredients list, which appears below the Nutrition Facts chart to determine whether you should bring this product along on your mission at all. When you read the ingredients list on some of your favorite "low-fat," "healthy" packaged foods, you'll likely find a laundry list of sugars, partially hydrogenated oils, artificial preservatives, and additives that should have you running for the produce aisle.

You may also find it helpful to consult a nutrition guide, internet or electronic calorie counter, or book to find listings of food values. You'll still have to do some math along the way, so keep your Recruit Field Journal handy. Within a few weeks of getting it right, you'll be much more familiar with appropriate portion sizes, and you'll learn to eyeball your meals to estimate how many grams of carbs, protein, and fats are found in the foods you normally eat.

The Big Picture

One more important word about consuming your daily target caloric intake.

Recruits often ask me whether they have to be completely accurate every single day. It's a good question, I hope you thought of it. Just as your body is smart enough to properly combine nutrients that come from different meals throughout the day rather than at one sitting, it's smart enough to adjust your metabolic rate based on your eating pattern rather than on what you do occasionally. You won't put on extra flab because once in a while you consume an entire bag of chips or eat an entire dessert; likewise, you won't take it off if you only eat well every now and then.

When what you eat, on average each week, reflects your optimal target energy intake and nutrient balance, you establish a pattern that helps your body adjust its rate of fat storage, fat burning, and muscle building. Slip off the narrow path once in a while and you won't interrupt the pattern; but making a habit of straying will put you right back where you started, Recruit. You may need to permit yourself an occasional decadence just to keep your sanity on this mission. If so, schedule it and keep track. Plan a specific day of liberty once a week or every couple of weeks when you can indulge in your favorite hedonistic habits and don't worry about the fat, sugar, nutrient balance, or anything else. Then discipline yourself and get back to training!

You now have a picture of how to eat and how much you need to eat to get started. Review your orders, Recruit, and remember that you will recalculate your nutrient requirements as you move toward your physique objectives. The formulas and guidelines you need are repeated in your Recruit Field Journal, so it should only take you a few minutes to calculate new requirements each time your body weight changes by at least 10 pounds or your activity level changes. Keep your data current. When you do, you will stay prepared to make steady, predictable progress toward your goals.

Summary of Orders

> **After calculating your daily target caloric intake, you will consume that required number of calories daily.**

> **You will balance your daily target caloric intake to include 1.4 grams of lean protein for every kilogram of your body weight, no more than 15% of your total calories from fat, and the balance of calories from low-GI carbs, including 25 to 30 grams of fiber.**

BRIEFING #6
Dietary Supplements

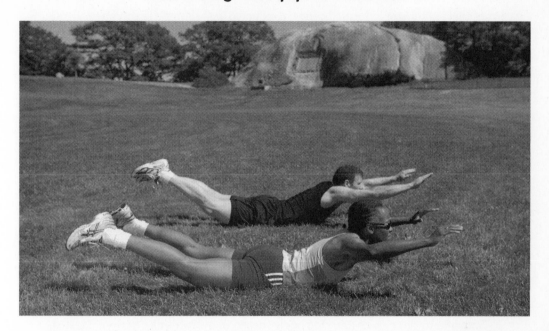

BEFORE WE EVEN BEGIN THE DISCUSSION, let's be clear, Recruit. The information on the appropriate use of dietary supplements is vast, so your orders here are only intended to provide you with some guidance on making good choices if you decide to use supplements. There is some introductory intel you need to have, and then you need to get smart on your own about what you might, and might not, need to use. So make sure you check the additional resources listed in the Reference section and expand your knowledge base.

For starters, just like with your food, learn to read labels. Just because some gorilla at your local gym swears by a popular meal replacement drink doesn't mean its ingredients are any better for you than a candy bar. Open your eyes! Even without any technical knowledge, your common sense should tell you that one-size-fits-all doses of roots, nuts, leaves, hormones, and enzymes can't be the right formula for every individual's optimal health and performance. Have the self-respect to think and act for yourself.

When considering any supplement, herb, or drug (even your prescriptions), your first thought should be: "What is the active ingredient, what does it do, and has it been proven effective in legitimate studies for my needs?" Clinical trials of any promising herb, drug, or additive are crucial for answering that question. Ideally, these trials should have been conducted by individuals and organizations that have no economic or political interest in any particular outcome. The results of the trials should have been written up in articles that are published in peer-reviewed journals. That means that legitimately educated people conducted well-designed experiments using live human beings at reputable institutions. They wrote down what they found out and what they think their findings mean. Then other reputable experts in the same field read about their studies in at least one of the hundreds of professional journals that get published every year. Those peers then discuss and decide whether the methods used and the results obtained were reliable. (Those that disagree may have written responses to the same journals pointing out the study's problems, so you can also read their opinions). Before any research is pronounced reliable, a few experts should have gotten similar results in different tests, on different subjects, and, over time, no one should have gotten really sick or died from using the product.

Sound complicated? Good call. It is complicated! That's why you can't just start swallowing pills and powders without thinking. It's also why the snake oil and magic elixir-makers assume that you'll never know any better than to buy most of the garbage they offer for sale. "Health" stores, Web sites, and fitness gurus pushing shelves of tree bark, animal sex hormones, fat burners, muscle builders, and miracle powders bet that you'll be dazzled by hype and too busy shopping to read.

You have to smarten up and stop being sucked in by words like "proven," "tested," "guaranteed," and "miracle" printed in large type on labels and store displays. Until you read the actual proof, it's all just smoke and mirrors. Science moves relatively slowly (just ask anyone with a serious disease), so claims of "new discoveries," "breakthroughs," and "secret ingredients" don't even merit a walk-through inspection until you can track down several peer-reviewed studies showing the claims are real.

To make things worse, even with legitimate science behind an ingredient and the endless babbling about "all natural" products, many of the items on your store shelves are simply inferior or ineffective. Need an example? You've probably heard of the promises of ginseng and seen the myriad of ginseng products advertised. Real ginseng does help boost athletic performance, energy levels, endurance, brain power, and physical recovery. Sounds great, right? Hold on a second. There are only three types of real ginseng in the world: panax ginseng and Sanchi or Tienchi ginseng, from China and Korea, and American ginseng. Controlled studies have shown legitimate and promising effects of ginseng supplementation using real ginseng herb standardized to deliver 200 mg per day of the effective ingredient, known as ginsenosides.

How Gullible Do You Have to Be?

In the mid 1990's a supplement called "Vitamin O" appeared in national newspaper ads and on Web sites. Its producers and distributors claimed that the solution of "stabilized oxygen molecules" in salt water, when taken orally, would purify the bloodstream, improve one's ability to metabolize nutrients, and detoxify the body. The supplement was allegedly developed in the '60's by a Dr. William F. Koch, and used by NASA to improve oxygen use by astronauts.

According to the ads, "Vitamin O' could treat or prevent everything from cancer and lung disease to memory loss and joint pain. The claims were backed by dozens of "testimonials" and "scientific and medical research."

The facts? Of course there is no Vitamin O. In 1999, the Federal Trade Commission reached a settlement with the product's marketers requiring them to stop claiming any health benefits from Vitamin O because:

> **no medical or scientific studies validate the product**

> **the supplement has no beneficial effect on human health**

> **the supplement wasn't even developed by Dr. Koch and was never used by NASA.**

Can you still get some? Of course. Since the product didn't actually harm anyone (it's just salt water), the FTC agreement could only require the company to stop making false claims. As long as the marketers' ads contain a disclaimer (even in tiny print) acknowledging their lack of science or validated testimonials, and once they paid the $375,000 in federal fines for consumer redress, they keep charging $20 an ounce for their saline solution!

So what's the problem? Just because you picked some ginseng plants doesn't mean that your handful of roots and leaves contains the right amount of the active ingredient. To be effective, herbs and other natural ingredients taken as supplements must be standardized so that every capsule, teaspoon, or drop delivers the precise, effective amount of the active ingredient. Reducing truckloads of imported roots and leaves into bottles on store shelves in which every capsule contains the correct amount of the herb's effective ingredient is a time-consuming, expensive process. The best-quality ginseng herbs, for example, only yield about 1 to 2% active ginsenosides. So what's the likelihood that every company-with-a-post-office-box address is spending the time and money to extract enough active ingredients from the plants and provide a standardized product in every package? Not likely. One analyst tested fifty-four "ginseng" products from store shelves and found that nearly 60% contained only small amounts—if any —ginsenosides.

The internationally renowned Colgan Institute for Sports Nutrition got similar results from several brands of "ginseng" tea. More recent random tests of 18 products found two of them high in contaminants or far less of the active ingredient than labeled. And that's the story on just one supplement! Most of the profit-hungry salesfolk are betting that you've only heard some word of mouth about any particular product, that you're willing to invest a few dollars in the promise of miracles, and that you have no idea what an effective ingredient is, let alone whether they put any in their bottle.

There are still more questions you need to ask before you take any supplement. Even if the stuff is real and its results are proven, how much are you supposed to take and is it appropriate for you? No matter which product you consider, you need to learn what dosage of the active ingredient has been shown effective and whether it has any potential side effects that might be relevant. If you choose a product that contains *some* of a supplement's active ingredient, but not as much as the amount that gave the promised results in trials, you're wasting your money and you won't achieve your objective.

Many substances are toxic in doses larger than the tested amounts or dangerous for people with certain conditions. Why, you might ask, would anyone take more than the effective dose? Good question. Some people decide that if a small dose of something can help them reach their goals, then a larger dose will speed the results. Here's a clue: Sleeping pills help you get to sleep, but too many can put you to sleep permanently. Some people assume that if the product is "natural" it's harmless. Clue: Poison ivy and arsenic are natural, but not harmless. Some people combine products with similar effects, either without thinking or because they think more is better. Clue: Tranquilizers and alcohol both calm you down; combining them can make you rest in peace. Hundreds of folks have shown up as statistics in the FDA's database of Adverse Events Reports, a listing of problems, illnesses, and deaths that were reported in connection with the use of dietary supplements. (This listing was discontinued in 1999 when the FDA decided its format wasn't terribly helpful for consumers. The government is currently working to develop a more informative system for presenting reliable information on supplements)

The FDA and several state governments continually consider legislation to try to save people from their own recklessness by limiting their access to various nutritional supplements. These efforts follow the logic from kindergarten when everyone's recess was cut short because of that one kid who kept breaking the rules. Fortunately for recruits who do use their brains, overreaching regulatory efforts have generally failed and you can still get effective supplements from reputable manufacturers. But that means that the snake oil salesmen also get to keep operating. Making smart choices is your responsibility. You have to learn where to turn for the right answers, and you have to stay knowledgeable about the products you choose.

How can you protect yourself? Learn all the effective ingredients for every supplement on the market, ask your dealer to show you the lab results from every manufacturer's products, and then choose the ones that contain what the labels say they do. That option should seem too complicated to you unless you have a great deal of free time, Recruit. Instead, you should also carefully consider your needs, look for objective information about supplements that can address those needs, identify a few manufacturers with consistently good reputations, and then stick with them for your supplies. Sound like a smarter plan? It should.

ConsumerLab.com is an independent testing company that provides information to help consumers and healthcare professionals evaluate health, wellness, and nutrition products. An online subscription for $24 per year gives you access to their results and lists of companies whose products they've approved. ConsumerLab.com gives its stamp of approval only after purchasing the product off the shelf, just as consumers would do, and using industry standard tests to determine that the product:

> **meets recognized quality standards.**

> **contains precisely what the label says it does.**

> **is free of contaminants.**

> **breaks down properly for use in the body, and**

> **contains the same identity, potency and purity in each unit of the product.**

If you call or write to most supplement companies, you'll get a part-time receptionist who hems and haws when you ask about the source or standardization of their ingredients or when you want to know exactly who has "proven" that their "breakthrough formula" is safe and effective. Your request to have additional information sent to you usually gets your address on their catalog mailing list but not much else. Do yourself a favor when you find these rogues—don't buy any of their products. At best, they won't work for you. At worst, you might wake up dead!

Companies such as Twinlab®, Nature's Herbs® (a Twinlab subsidiary), Puritan's Pride®, Vitamin World®, and others have well-established reputations for producing supplements and herbals that contain quality ingredients and the effective dose of each active ingredient. Check with ConsumerLab.com or refer to other sources listed in the Reference section if you choose to use nutritional supplements.

Remember this: Supplements are substances that boost the solid nutritional foundation you must have already established. No supplement can deliver miracle results if you don't do your work on the training field and at the dinner table. If you're looking for enhanced brain functioning, higher energy, bigger muscles, faster running, or better performance in bed, start by eating properly, drinking your water, getting enough sleep (at least 8 hours a night), and training consistently. Then, and only then, if you need a little help, consider supplementing. When you do, you must review your specific situation. You must determine how much you need to take, how often, and for how long. You will base that decision, at minimum, on your goals, your training level, your gender, your body weight, and your health history. And then you have to learn whether any supplement is potentially dangerous for you.

So, before you start swallowing pills and powders to enhance your health or physical performance:

1) **Take a hard look at your nutrition, training, and sleeping habits. If they aren't optimal, no amount of supplementation is going to get you to your objective. Go back to the K.I.S.S. rule. Fix the basics first, Recruit.**

2) **Educate yourself about the effects—both positive and negative—of everything that catches your attention in newspaper articles, TV ads, your gym's juice bar, and health food store displays. Be honest and realistic about your health history and lifestyle habits. Read the studies and reports, not just the propaganda from the manufacturer, salesman, or weight room staff.**

3) **Tell your doc about any supplements you're considering or are already taking. Some herbs and increased doses of other vitamins and minerals can interact with prescription medicines. And be advised, Recruit, you also have to educate yourself about your doc. Most general practitioners are not up to speed on nutrition, sports supplementation, or performance. If you're lucky, your doc is open-minded, honest about knowledge gaps, and willing to get smart or refer you to someone who is. If your doc is an old-school drone who either ignores the details because she thinks all sports supplements are harmless or recommends against using anything—ever—because he thinks all supplements are worthless, get a new doc. You don't need the dead weight on your team.**

4) **Be patient. No worthwhile changes happen overnight, and there are no legitimate supplements that work miracles. Your body has to incorporate every new substance into its systems and, in some cases, clear out negative or ineffective substances before you'll see positive changes. That usually takes months, not days. The weak-minded folks that rave about how much stronger, faster, smarter, or leaner they were after only a few days of taking a magic potion are either trying to sell something or experiencing a placebo effect—improvements that**

occur just because you believe you've swallowed a magic potion. Be patient and realistic, Recruit. Some improvements are purely metabolic or systemic and can only be detected in lab tests; ask your doc for help with checking on your progress. Other positive effects that you will see or feel may take six months or more to occur, so give it time.

Use your brain, read your labels, correct your basic habits, and then consider supplements that might further your goals. When you decide to help boost your performance, don't be swindled. You'll find more sources for reliable supplement information and purchasing guidance in the Reference section (page 143).

Summary of Orders

> When considering whether to include nutritional supplements in your mission plan, you will first ensure that you are training hard, eating well, and getting enough sleep.

> Then think about what you're trying to accomplish with supplements and look for reliable information about which supplements, the proper dosage and forms, and the best manufacturers than can help with your goals.

BOOT CAMP ABS

the beginning

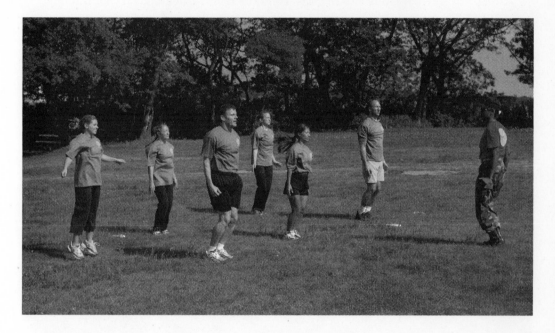

Welcome to a brand new day, Recruit. You've learned some new things about the most complicated machine in the warehouse, your body. You've gathered the information you need about how and what to feed it. And your training plans provide a map to putting it through the paces that will start to help you tune it up.

Optimal performance. Desirable appearance. Goal achievement. Theyy're all on the horizon.

"What now?"

In case you've forgotten where you've been, here's the full summary of your orders on nutrition:

DIRECT ORDER #1: Eat every 3 to 4 hours.

DIRECT ORDER #2: Consume primarily low-GI carbs.

DIRECT ORDER #3: Get 25 to 30 grams of fiber daily.

DIRECT ORDER #4: Consume lean, high-quality protein.

DIRECT ORDER #5: Consume small amounts of fats.

DIRECT ORDER #6: Emphasize essential and monounsaturated fats from cold-water fatty fish and pure vegetable oils.

DIRECT ORDER #7: Drink 8 to 16 glasses of water daily (depending on your training schedule).

DIRECT ORDER #8: Consider nutritional supplements only after you lay a solid foundation of balanced eating, solid training, and quality sleep; then get the best information you can find before purchasing the best quality supplements you can find.

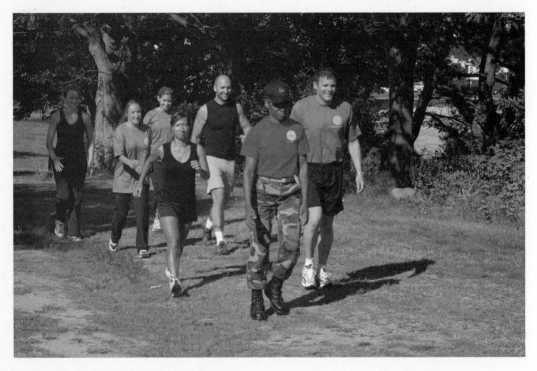

To review your training tasks:

You will provide overload to your muscles by starting with an appropriate volume and intensity of work to induce some hypertrophy (muscle fiber growth), and you will gradually increase that overload to keep the positive changes coming. On this mission that will mean ab training four days a week. In addition, on your own, you will work your other muscles three to five days each week.

You will include aerobic work to speed up your metabolism, improve your cardiovascular endurance, and help burn the body fat that otherwise covers up all that hypertrophy. This mission's cardio work will be scheduled on three days each week.

And to keep yourself honest, you will monitor your nutrition intake by completing your Nutrition Logs daily and you will check off successful completion of each day's work on the Training Plans found in your Recruit Field Journal.

Those are your orders. Execution is up to you. Only one command remains, Recruit.

Forward, MARCH!

reference section

Calculating Nutrient Balance Requirements for High-Performance Athletes

Endurance Athletes

Those who participate in high-level endurance training lasting more than 90 minutes daily and who do not require specific changes to body weight should skip the calculation of target daily caloric intake and use the following amounts for calculating their target daily intake of each nutrient:

> **target carb grams daily: 8 to 10 g per kg body weight**

> **target protein grams daily: 1.5 g per kg body weight**

> **target fat daily: 20 to 35% of total daily caloric intake**

Power and Strength Athletes

Those who use heavy resistance training for greater power and strength and who do not require specific changes to body weight should skip the calculation of target daily caloric intake and use the following amounts for calculating their target daily intake of each nutrient:

> **target carb grams daily: 5 to 6 g per kg of body weight**

> **target protein grams daily: 1.7 to 1.8 g per kg body weight**

> **target fat daily: 15 to 20% of total daily caloric intake**

Additional Nutrition Information

Nutritional Composition of Foods

> **Netzer, Corinne, "The Complete Book of Food Counts,"** 6th Ed., Dell Publishing Company, 2003.

> **USDA National Nutrient Database:** http://www.nal.usda.gov/fnic/food-comp/search/

> **Fast Food Finder, from Olen Publishing, Inc., Minnesota.** A comprehensive Web site search tool for information on the composition of foods from the most popular fast food restaurants based on the book "Fast Food Facts" published by the Minnesota Office of the Attorney General. http://www.olen.com/food/

> **Glycemic Index of Foods, Revised International Table of Glycemic Index (GI) and Glycemic Load (GL) Values, 2002.** http://diabetes.about.com/library/mendosagi/ngilists.htm

Choosing Supplements

> **Gatorade Sports Science Institute, Sports Science Center.** Several articles from leading nutritionists evaluating some of the most popular dietary supplements, their safety and effectiveness. http://www.gssiweb.com/sportssciencecenter/ (Choose "Sports Science Topics" for most purposes.)

> **ConsumerLab.com.** A subscription-based Web site reporting independent lab test results for vitamin, mineral, herbal, and performance supplements from many different manufacturers along with a comprehensive encyclopedia of natural products with their purposes, effectiveness, and potential side effects. http://www.consumerlab.com/

Rating Other Nutritional Information

> **Tufts University Nutrition Navigator.** An online rating and review guide of Web sites that provide nutrition information and diet plans. Sites are reviewed by the nutritionists of Boston's prestigious Tufts University School of Nutrition Science and Policy using criteria developed by some of the leading U.S. and Canadian nutrition experts. Find out which sites contain accurate and trustworthy advice. http://www.navigator.tufts.edu/

Reference Citations

> Chapter notes with support for the facts, claims, and scientific evidence cited throughout this book can be found online at the FitBoot web site: http://www.fitboot.com/bootcampabsnotes.shtml

recruit field journal

Data Locations

Fitness Assessment Results Log

RECORD THE RESULTS of your initial fitness assessment on the chart located here. In the last column, circle the skill level designation you earned for each event as listed on the Fitness Assessment Scoring Instructions (page 154). As described earlier, you will score your performance events and choose the appropriate training exercises using the shooter designations: Marksman, Sharpshooter, or Expert. Your vital signs and body composition measurements are assigned within the range of: Green Light, On Target, Yellow Zone, or Red Zone so you can gauge whether you need to include improvement goals or work to maintain your current level.

Once you start training, you will check your progress and update your scores using these charts each time you repeat the Fitness Assessment.

Initial Fitness Assessment Results

Date: _____

DATA	RESULT	SKILL DESIGNATION
Age		
Height	"	
Weight	lbs.	*(See Height/Weight Chart, p. 155)* *Green Light* On Target Red Zone
Resting Heart Rate	b.p.m	Green Light On Target Red Zone
Blood Pressure		Green Light On Target Red Zone
Body Composition Measures Using: (circle one) BIA Circumference BMI Waist-to-Hip		Green Light On Target Yellow Zone Red Zone
Ground Zero Estimate	Pushes Off Deck	Green Light On Target Yellow Zone Red Zone
Timed Curl-ups 1:00		*(See Fitness Test Assessment Chart, p. 154)* Green Light On Target Yellow Zone Red Zone

Fitness Assessment Progress Results
End of Week 4
Date: _____

DATA	RESULT	SKILL DESIGNATION
Age		
Height	"	
Weight	lbs.	*(See Height/Weight Chart, p. 155)* On Target Red Zone
Resting Heart Rate	b.p.m	Green Light On Target Red Zone
Blood Pressure		Green Light On Target Red Zone
Body Composition Measures Using: (circle one) BIA Circumference BMI Waist-to-Hip		Green Light On Target Yellow Zone Red Zone
Ground Zero Estimate	Pushes Off Deck	Green Light On Target Yellow Zone Red Zone
Timed Curl-ups 2:00		*(See Fitness Test Assessment Chart, p. 154)* Green Light On Target Yellow Zone Red Zone

Fitness Assessment Progress Results
End of Week 8

Date: _____

DATA	RESULT	SKILL DESIGNATION
Age		
Height	"	
Weight	lbs.	*(See Height/Weight Chart, p. 155)* On Target Red Zone
Resting Heart Rate	b.p.m	Green Light On Target Red Zone
Blood Pressure		Green Light On Target Red Zone
Body Composition Measures Using: (circle one) BIA Circumference BMI Waist-to-Hip		Green Light On Target Yellow Zone Red Zone
Ground Zero Estimate	Pushes Off Deck	Green Light On Target Yellow Zone Red Zone
Timed Curl-ups 2:00		*(See Fitness Test Performance Scoring Chart, p. 154)* Green Light On Target Yellow Zone Red Zone

Nutrition Requirements Log

MARK THE RESULTS of your nutrition requirements calculations from the worksheets. Do it in pencil, Recruit, so you can update them as you reach your goals and as your needs change.

Daily Target Caloric Intake _____

Target Fat Intake: _____ calories, _____ grams, <u>15</u>%

Target Protein Intake: _____ calories, _____ grams, _____ %

Target Carbohydrate Intake: _____ calories, _____ grams, _____%

(remember to include 25 to 30 grams of fiber daily)

Fitness Assessment Scoring Instructions

Height/Weight Chart

Although no research supports a specific "perfect" weight for a given individual, there are ranges of "normal" or desirable body weights for men and women at given ages and heights. These norms have been derived from population data collected for more than 100 years, primarily by insurance companies, and have been adopted and modified to account for health-related guidelines given by the American Heart Association. We will use the 1959 values published by Metropolitan Life Insurance Company. The ranges were revised in 1983, but the later values included a 12- to14 pound increase in body weight for shorter individuals. The American Heart Association and National Institutes of Health identify a major problem with these adjusted ranges: "Such increased body weight may contribute to high blood pressure, hypercholesterolemia, and glucose intolerance or similar risk factors, apart from the impact of weight on mortality."

To estimate your frame size, wrap the thumb and middle finger of your right hand around your left wrist. If you can barely touch the tip of your middle finger with your thumb, you are large framed; if you can touch anywhere from the fingernail to the first joint you are medium framed; if you can reach farther than the first joint, you are small framed.

If you're within the designated range, you're On Target. Anything above the designated range for your age and gender or more than 5 pounds below the range puts you in the Red Zone. However, you must also consider your body composition score when you consider the height/weight chart. If you fall near the top or above the designated range, adjust your assessment to reflect your body composition score.

WOMEN

HEIGHT	SMALL FRAME	MEDIUM FRAME	LARGE FRAME
4'8"	92-98 lbs.	96-107 lbs.	104-119 lbs.
4'9"	94-101	98-110	106-122
4'10"	96-104	101-113	109-125
4'11""	99-107	104-116	112-128
5'0"	102-110	107-119	115-131
5'1"	105-113	110-122	118-134
5'2"	108-116	113-126	121-138
5'3"	111-119	116-130	125-142
5'4"	114-123	120-135	129-146
5'5"	118-127	124-139	133-150
5'6"	121-131	128-143	137-154
5'7"	126-135	132-147	141-158
5'8"	130-140	136-151	145-163
5'9"	134-144	140-155	149-168
5'11"	138-148	144-159	153-173

MEN

HEIGHT	SMALL FRAME	MEDIUM FRAME	LARGE FRAME
5'1"	112-120 lbs.	118-129 lbs.	126-141 lbs.
5'2"	115-123	121-133	129-144
5'3"	118-126	124-136	132-148
5'4"	121-129	127-139	135-152
5'5"	124-133	130-143	138-156
5'6"	128-137	134-147	142-161
5'7"	132-141	138-152	147-166
5'8"	136-145	142-156	151-170
5'9"	140-150	146-160	155-174
5'10"	144-154	150-165	159-179
5'11"	148-158	154-170	164-184
6'0"	152-162	158-175	168-189
6'1"	156-167	162-180	173-194
6'2"	160-171	167-185	178-199
6'3"	164-175	172-190	182-204

Adapted from Metropolitan Life Insurance Company. New weight standards for men and women.
Stat Bull Metropol Life Insur Co 1959;40:14.

Body Composition Ranges

BIA (Bioelectrical Impedance Analysis)

If you have had your body fat estimated using BIA, use the following chart to interpret your score.

% BODY-FAT RATIOS	
WOMEN	
17-22%	Green Light *Note: less than 10% body fat for women is Red Zone, for health reasons (See explanation of body composition and storage fat in opening section on Fitness Assessment before beginning program).*
22-25%	On Target
25-29%	Yellow Zone
29-35%	Red Zone *Note: above 35% is extreme Red Zone (read: obesity). Get to work, Recruit!*
MEN	
10-15%	Green Light *Note: less than 5% body fat for males is Red Zone, for health reasons (See explanation of body composition and storage fat in opening section on Fitness Assessment before beginning program).*
15-18%	On Target
18-20%	Yellow Zone
20-25%	Red Zone *Note: above 25% is extreme Red Zone (read: obesity). Get out of there, Recruit!*

BMI (Body Mass Index)

If you have used BMI to estimate body composition, use the following chart to interpret your score.

BMI RESULTS

WOMEN	
25 or below	Green Light
25.8-27.2	On Target
27.3-29.9	Yellow Zone
30+	Red Zone
MEN	
26 or below	Green Light
26.4-27.7	On Target
27.8-29.9	Yellow Zone
30+	Red Zone

WAIST-TO-HIP RATIO

If you have used Weight-to-Height to estimate the location of body fat, use the following scores.

The higher the number, the higher your estimated health risks.

WAIST-TO-HIP RATIO

WOMEN		
.79 or lower	Pear	On Target
.80 or higher	Apple	Red Zone
MEN		
.99 or below	Pear	On Target
1.0 or higher	Apple	Red Zone

Fitness Performance Scores

ABDOMINAL STRENGTH AND ENDURANCE

GROUND-ZERO ESTIMATE

WOMEN AND MEN

appx. 8" or less from the ground	Green Light
appx. 8-12" from the ground	On Target
appx 12-18" from the ground	Yellow Zone
higher than 18" from the ground	Red Zone

TIMED CURL-UPS (1:00) (Initial Assessment)

WOMEN AND MEN

50-60	Green Light
40-49	On Target
30-39	Yellow Zone
29 or fewer	Red Zone

TIMED CURL-UPS (2:00) (Progress Checks)

WOMEN AND MEN

90-100	Green Light
75-89	On Target
60-74	Yellow Zone
59 or fewer	Red Zone

Nutrition Requirements Worksheets

USE THIS WORKSHEET TO CALCULATE your nutrition requirements for mission launch. You will recalculate your requirements and record the new amounts, if changes in body weight are part of your goals, each time your weight changes by at least 10 pounds. Use a pencil so you can reuse this worksheet! You will record your requirements on the charts that follow.

Estimated Daily Energy Expenditure Rate (RDEER):

WOMEN:

**661 + (weight in lbs. x 4.38) + (height in inches x 4.33)
– (age in years x 4.7) = _____RMR**

MEN:

**67 + (weight. in lbs. x 6.24) + (height in inches x 12.7)
– (age in years x 6.8) = _____RMR**

Now multiply your RMR by one of the following values to account for your daily activity level as follows.

ACTIVITY MULTIPLIER CHART

ACTIVITY LEVEL	MULTIPLY RMR BY:
currently inactive and crash dieted in the past	.9
currently inactive but never crash dieted	1.2
exercising 3 days/week, at least 1 hour, no physically demanding daily activities	1.3
exercising 4-5 days/week, at least 1 hour	1.5
exercising 5-6 days/week, at least 1 hour	1.7
exercising daily, more than 1 hour, training for very high endurance sports, and/or physically demanding, continuous work daily	1.9

Result = _____calories Daily Energy Expenditure Rate (DEER)

Calculate any required adjustment to your DEER to determine your Target Daily Caloric Intake

NO WEIGHT CHANGE REQUIRED	DEER = TARGET DAILY CALORIC INTAKE
Weight loss required	DEER x .3 = _____caloric adjustment
	if result is higher than 500, use 500 as caloric adjustment
	DEER – caloric adjustment = _____ Target Daily Caloric Intake
Weight gain required	DEER x .3 = _____caloric adjustment
	if result is higher than 500, use 500 as caloric adjustment
	DEER + caloric adjustment = _____ Target Daily Caloric Intake

Nutrient Balance Requirements

Carbohydrate Requirements

(*Note: Expert-level endurance athletes, see Reference Section)

**Daily Target Caloric Intake –
(Target protein calories + Target fat calories) =
_____Target carb calories**

Target carb calories x 4 = _____Target carb grams

**Target carb calories ÷ Daily Target Caloric Intake =
____% of calories from carbs**

Protein Requirements

*(*Note: Power and strength athletes training more than 2 hours daily, see Reference Section)*

Body weight ÷ 2.2 = _____ kg body weight

kg body weight x 1.4 = _____Target protein grams

Target protein grams x 4 = _____Target protein calories

Target protein calories ÷ Daily Target Caloric Intake = _____% of calories from protein

Fat Requirements:

*(*Note: Expert-level endurance athletes, see Reference Section)*

Daily Target Caloric Intake x .15 = _____Target fat calories

Target fat calories ÷ 9 = _____Target fat grams

RESTING HEART RATE CHART

40-65 b.p.m.	Green Light
66-100 b.p.m	On Target
100+ b.p.m.	Red Zone

DAILY NUTRITION LOG

Day of the Week: _____   **Date:** _____

MEAL	FOOD	CALORIES	G CARBS	G PROTEIN	G FAT
Breakfast					
Snack					
Lunch					

MEAL	FOOD	CALORIES	G CARBS	G PROTEIN	G FAT
Snack					
Dinner					
Snack					
TOTAL DAILY INTAKE					

The Training Plans

TIME TO GET YOUR WORK DONE, RECRUIT.

You can decide to work your abs before or after other muscle groups, but make sure to complete the assigned ab routine in one sitting (don't sprinkle ab exercises throughout your regular routine or use them to fill rest periods—that practice tends to give the abs too much recovery time between sets as opposed to the work you do for your other muscles). Your ab routines are generally written as series of circuits, so complete the designated number of repetitions for each exercise, rest for 30 to 40 seconds, and then complete the series again for the specified number of sets.

Listed here are 8-week training plans for each skill level. Stay with your unit, Recruit! Stick to the exercises in your skill level for abdominal strength/endurance. Although you will check your progress in Week 4, you will not change your exercise skill level until you complete Week 8 to ensure that you fully adapt, physically and mentally, to proper exercise technique and the increasing training volume.

If you move to the next skill level after completing your 8-week program, march forward to the training plan for that new skill designation. If you are not yet proficient enough to advance, return to Week 4 at your current skill level, review the descriptions and training advisories for each exercise, work to improve your mental focus and physical technique, and check your progress again in four more weeks.

Those starting at Expert level, complete your training plan, then return to Week 1 of any other skill level and add 4 to 6 reps to each exercise as you navigate another 8 weeks.

The Recipe: Sets and Reps

Your training plans list the number of sets and repetitions ("reps") you will perform for each exercise. You salty vets who've trained in the past and are familiar with how sets and reps are listed in training plans, stand at ease while I brief the raw recruits.

The number of times you must perform an exercise without resting is the number of reps required. When you perform the required number of reps you've completed one set for that exercise. Your training plans list the number of sets required times the number of reps, with the amount of rest time, if any, listed in parentheses:

For example:

Circuits (groups) of exercises followed by a REST command.

> **> Circuit**

> **> Reverse crunches—2 x 10**

> **> Flutter kicks—2 x 10**

> **> Crunches—2 x 10**

> **> REST :15**

You will perform one set of 1 repetition of each of these exercises in sequence, you will then rest for 15 seconds, and you will perform the second set of each exercise in sequence.

Required number of reps at a specified effort level with recovery activity in parentheses.

> **> Running Hills—4 x uphill (moderate run down)**

You will run uphill one time, return to the bottom of the hill at a moderate pace, and run uphill again, repeating for 4 uphill trips.

Timed or distance exercises listing the required number of sets times the distance, if applicable, at a specified time or exertion level with rest time or recovery activity, if any, in parentheses.

> **> Timed Curl-ups: 1 x :90 (:60)**

You will perform the timed curl-ups exercise for 90 seconds continuously (brief 2-3 second rests are permitted so long as you resume moving and finish your 90 second drill). You will then rest for 60 seconds.

> **> Interval Sprints: 2 x 25 yds @ fast (walk 25 yds)**

You will run one sprint, 25 yards long, at what you perceive as a fast pace. You will walk for 25 yards and then run another 25 yards at a fast pace.]Unless otherwise indicated, perform all exercises at moderate pace, keeping the count— either in your head or out loud—just like a military march cadence: "1, 2, 3,—1 1, 2 , 3,—2".

Permission is granted for a BRIEF pause between exercises (except in Circuits) to catch your breath and take a drink of water when necessary. You will not eyeball the area. You will not wait until your heart rate returns to couch-lounging level. You will not waste time flapping your gums with your training buddy or with the strangers in the park who marvel at your progress and want to know your secret. Tell friends and observers to "fall in!" next to you and begin. Better yet, tell them to buy the book and then you can all meet every morning in the park and get some work done!

Let's get moving!

MARKSMAN

Marksman Week 1

TRAINING DAY 1	TRAINING DAY 2	TRAINING DAY 3	TRAINING DAY 4
Circuit: 2 x 10 Superman Reverse crunches Crunches Lying sidebends REST :30	Circuit: 2 x 10 The Swimmer Tiltups-knees bent Legs up Crunches Alternate leg crunches REST :30	Circuit: 2 x 10 Superman Reverse crunches Crunches Lying sidebends REST :30	Circuit: 2 x 10 The Swimmer Tiltups-knees bent Legs up Crunches Alternate leg crunches REST :30
Power walk 40:00	Distance Run 1 mile	Power walk 40:00	

Marksman Week 2

TRAINING DAY 1	TRAINING DAY 2	TRAINING DAY 3	TRAINING DAY 4
Circuit: 2 x 12 Superman Reverse crunches Crunches Lying sidebends REST :30	Circuit: 2 x 12 The Swimmer Tiltups-knees bent Legs up Crunches Alternate leg crunches REST :30	Circuit: 2 x 12 Superman Reverse crunches Crunches Lying sidebends REST :30	Timed curl-ups 2 x :60 (:60)
Power walk 40:00		Power walk 40:00	Distance Run 1 mile

Marksman Week 3

TRAINING DAY 1	TRAINING DAY 2	TRAINING DAY 3	TRAINING DAY 4
Circuit: 3x 10 Superman Reverse crunches Crunches Lying sidebends REST :30	Circuit: 3x 10 The Swimmer Tiltups-knees bent Legs up Crunches Alternate leg crunches REST :30	Circuit: 3x 10 Superman Reverse crunches Crunches Lying sidebends REST :30	Timed curl-ups 1 x :90 (:60) 1 x :60 (:60) 1 x :30
Power walk 40:00	Distance Run 1.5 mile	Power walk 40:00	

Marksman Week 4

TRAINING DAY 1	TRAINING DAY 2	TRAINING DAY 3	TRAINING DAY 4
Circuit: 2x 15 Superman Reverse crunches Crunches Lying sidebends REST :30	Circuit: 3x 12 The Swimmer Tiltups-knees bent Legs up Crunches Alternate leg crunches REST :30	Circuit: 2x 15 Superman Reverse crunches Crunches Lying sidebends REST :30	**PROGRESS CHECK**
Interval Sprints 2x 25 yds @easy (walk 25 yds) 2 x 25 yds@moderate (walk 25 yds) 2 x 25 yds @fast (walk 25 yds) 2 x 50 yds @moderate (walk 25 yds) 1 x 50 yds @fast (walk 25 yds) 1 x 75 yds @moderate (walk 25 yds) 1 x 75 yds@fast (walk 25 yds)		Interval Sprints 2x 25 yds @easy (walk 25 yds) 2 x 25 yds@moderate (walk 25 yds) 2 x 25 yds @fast (walk 25 yds) 2 x 50 yds @moderate (walk 25 yds) 1 x 50 yds @fast (walk 25 yds) 1 x 75 yds @moderate (walk 25 yds) 1 x 75 yds@fast (walk 25 yds)	Distance Run 2 miles Ground zero Estimate Timed curl-ups 1 x :60

Marksman Week 5

TRAINING DAY 1	TRAINING DAY 2	TRAINING DAY 3	TRAINING DAY 4
Circuit: 2x 15 Superman Reverse crunches Crunches Lying sidebends REST :30	Circuit: 3x 12 The Swimmer Tiltups-knees bent Legs up Crunches Alternate leg crunches REST :30	Circuit: 2x 15 Superman Reverse crunches Crunches Lying sidebends REST :30	Circuit: 2x 15 The Swimmer Tiltups-knees bent Legs up Crunches Alternate leg crunches REST :30
Interval Sprints 3x 25 yds @moderate (walk 25 yds) 3 x 25 yds@fast (walk 25 yds) 1 x 50 yds @easy (walk 25 yds) 1 x 50 yds @moderate (walk 25 yds) 1 x 50 yds @fast (walk 25 yds) 1 x 75 yds @moderate (walk 25 yds) 2 x 25 yds@fast (walk 25 yds)		Interval Sprints 3x 25 yds @moderate (walk 25 yds) 3 x 25 yds@fast (walk 25 yds) 1 x 50 yds @easy (walk 25 yds) 1 x 50 yds @moderate (walk 25 yds) 1 x 50 yds @fast (walk 25 yds) 1 x 75 yds @moderate (walk 25 yds) 2 x 25 yds@fast (walk 25 yds)	Distance Run 2.5 miles

Marksman Week 6

TRAINING DAY 1	TRAINING DAY 2	TRAINING DAY 3	TRAINING DAY 4
Circuit: 3x 15 Superman Reverse crunches Crunches Lying sidebends REST :30	Circuit: 3x 15 The Swimmer Tiltups-knees bent Legs up Crunches Alternate leg crunches REST :30	Circuit: 3x 15 Superman Reverse crunches Crunches Lying sidebends REST :30	Distance Run 2.5 miles
Power Walk 45:00		Power Walk 45:00	Timed curl-ups 1 x 2:00 (:90) 1 x :90 (:90) 1 x :60 (:60) 2 x :30 (:30)

Marksman Week 7

TRAINING DAY 1	TRAINING DAY 2	TRAINING DAY 3	TRAINING DAY 4
Circuit: 4x 12	Circuit: 4x 12	Circuit: 4x 12	Circuit: 2x 15
Superman	The Swimmer	Superman	The Swimmer
Reverse crunches	Tiltups-knees bent	Reverse crunches	Tiltups-knees bent
Crunches	Legs up Crunches	Crunches	Legs up Crunches
Lying sidebends	Alternate leg crunches	Lying sidebends	Alternate leg crunches
REST :30	REST :30	REST :30	REST :30
Interval Sprints 4x 25 yds @moderate (walk 25 yds) 2 x 25 yds@fast (walk 25 yds) 2 x 50 yds @easy (walk 25 yds) 1 x 75 yds @moderate (walk 25 yds) 1 x 50 yds @fast (walk 25 yds) 1 x 75 yds @moderate (walk 25 yds) 2 x 25 yds@fast (walk 25 yds)		Interval Sprints 4x 25 yds @moderate (walk 25 yds) 2 x 25 yds@fast (walk 25 yds) 2 x 50 yds @easy (walk 25 yds) 1 x 75 yds @moderate (walk 25 yds) 1 x 50 yds @fast (walk 25 yds) 1 x 75 yds @moderate (walk 25 yds) 2 x 25 yds@fast (walk 25 yds)	Distance Run 3 miles

BOOT CAMP ABS

Marksman Week 8

TRAINING DAY 1	TRAINING DAY 2	TRAINING DAY 3	TRAINING DAY 4
Circuit: 4x 15 Superman Reverse crunches Crunches Lying sidebends REST :30	Circuit: 4x 15 The Swimmer Tiltups-knees bent Legs up Crunches Alternate leg crunches REST :30	Circuit: 4x 15 Superman Reverse crunches Crunches Lying sidebends REST :30	**PROGRESS CHECK**
			Ground zero estimate
Interval Sprints 3x 25 yds @moderate (walk 25 yds) 4x 25 yds@fast (walk 25 yds) 2 x 50 yds @moderate (walk 25 yds) 2 x 50 yds @fast (walk 25 yds) 2 x 75 yds @moderate (walk 25 yds) 1 x 100 yds @fast 2 x 25 yds@fast (walk 25 yds)	Power walk	Interval Sprints 3x 25 yds @moderate (walk 25 yds) 4x 25 yds@fast (walk 25 yds) 2 x 50 yds @moderate (walk 25 yds) 2 x 50 yds @fast (walk 25 yds) 2 x 75 yds @moderate (walk 25 yds) 1 x 100 yds @fast 2 x 25 yds@fast (walk 25 yds)	Timed curl-ups 1 x 2:00
			Distance Run 3 miles

SHARPSHOOTER

Sharpshooter Week 1

TRAINING DAY 1	TRAINING DAY 2	TRAINING DAY 3	TRAINING DAY 4
Circuit: 2 x 12 Superman Reverse crunches 4 count crunches Lying sidebends REST :30	Circuit: 2 x 12 The Swimmer Tiltups-knees bent 6 count crunches Legs up Crunches REST :30 Distance Run 1 mile	Circuit: 2 x 12 Superman Reverse crunches 4 count crunches Lying sidebends REST :30	Circuit: 2 x 12 The Swimmer Tiltups-knees bent 6 count crunches Legs up Crunches REST :30

Sharpshooter Week 2

TRAINING DAY 1	TRAINING DAY 2	TRAINING DAY 3	TRAINING DAY 4
Circuit: 2 x 15 Superman Reverse crunches 4 count crunches Lying sidebends REST :30	Circuit: 2 x 15 The Swimmer Tiltups-knees bent Legs up Crunches Alternate leg crunches REST :30	Circuit: 2 x 15 Superman Reverse crunches 4 count crunches Lying sidebends REST :30	Timed curl-ups 1 x :90(:60) 1 x :60 (:60) 1 x :30 Distance Run 1 mile

Sharpshooter Week 3

TRAINING DAY 1	TRAINING DAY 2	TRAINING DAY 3	TRAINING DAY 4
Circuit: 3x 12 Superman Flutter kicks Tiltups- legs straight Legs up crunches REST :30	Circuit: 3x 12 The Swimmer 4 count crunches Alternate leg crunches REST :30	Circuit: 3x 12 Superman Flutter kicks Tiltups- legs straight Legs up crunches REST :30	Timed curl-ups 1 x :90 (:60) 1 x :60 (:60) 1 x :30
	Distance Run 1.5 mile		

Sharpshooter Week 4

TRAINING DAY 1	TRAINING DAY 2	TRAINING DAY 3	TRAINING DAY 4
Circuit: 3x 15 Superman Flutter kicks Tiltups- legs straight Legs up crunches REST :30	Circuit: 3x 12 The Swimmer 4 count crunches Alternate leg crunches REST :30	Circuit: 3x 15 Superman Flutter kicks Tiltups- legs straight Legs up crunches REST :30	**PROGRESS CHECK**
			Distance Run 2 miles
			Ground zero Estimate
			Timed curl-ups 1 x :60

Sharpshooter Week 5

TRAINING DAY 1	TRAINING DAY 2	TRAINING DAY 3	TRAINING DAY 4
Circuit: 3x 15 Superman Reverse crunches 6 count crunches Lying sidebends REST :30	Circuit: 3x 12 The Swimmer Tiltups-knees bent 4 count crunches Legs up Crunches REST :30	Circuit: 3x 15 Superman Reverse crunches 6 count crunches Lying sidebends REST :30	Circuit: 3x 15 The Swimmer Tiltups-knees straight Legs up Crunches Alternate leg crunches REST :30
			Distance Run 2.5 miles

Sharpshooter Week 6

TRAINING DAY 1	TRAINING DAY 2	TRAINING DAY 3	TRAINING DAY 4
Circuit: 4x 12 Superman Reverse crunches 6 count crunches Lying sidebends REST :30	Circuit: 4x 15 The Swimmer Tiltups-knees bent 4 count crunches Legs up Crunches REST :30	Circuit: 4x 12 Superman Reverse crunches 6 count crunches Lying sidebends REST :30	Distance Run 2.5 miles
			Timed curl-ups 1 x 2:00 (:90) 1 x :90 (:90) 1 x :60 (:60) 2 x :30 (:30)

Sharpshooter Week 7

TRAINING DAY 1	TRAINING DAY 2	TRAINING DAY 3	TRAINING DAY 4
Circuit: 4x 12 Superman Flutter kicks 6 count crunches Legs up crunches REST :30	Circuit: 4x 15 The Swimmer Tiltups-knees bent 4 count crunches Legs up Crunches REST :30	Circuit: 4x 12 Superman Flutter kicks 6 count crunches Legs up crunches REST :30	Circuit: 4x 15 The Swimmer Tiltups-knees bent Legs up Crunches Alternate leg crunches REST :30
			Distance Run 3 miles

Sharpshooter Week 8

TRAINING DAY 1	TRAINING DAY 2	TRAINING DAY 3	TRAINING DAY 4
Circuit: 2x 20 Superman Tilt ups—legs straight 4 count crunches Lying sidebends REST :30	Circuit: 4x 15 The Swimmer Tiltups-knees bent Legs up Crunches Alternate leg crunches REST :30	Circuit: 2x 20 Superman Tilt ups—legs straight 4 count crunches Lying sidebends REST :30	**PROGRESS CHECK**
			Ground zero
			Timed curl-ups 1 x 2:00
			Distance Run 3 miles

EXPERT

Expert Week 1

TRAINING DAY 1	TRAINING DAY 2	TRAINING DAY 3	TRAINING DAY 4
Circuit: 2 x 12 Superman Reverse crunches Tilt-ups—legs straight Legs up crunches REST :30	Circuit: 2 x 12 The Swimmer Lying sidebends 6 count crunches V-sits REST :30	Circuit: 2 x 12 Superman Reverse crunches Tilt-ups—legs straight Legs up crunches REST :30	Circuit: 2 x 12 The Swimmer Lying sidebends 6 count crunches V-sits REST :30
Distance Run 1.5 miles	Distance Run 1.5 mile	Distance Run 1.5 miles	

Expert Week 2

TRAINING DAY 1	TRAINING DAY 2	TRAINING DAY 3	TRAINING DAY 4
Circuit: 3 x 12 Superman Reverse crunches Tilt-ups—legs straight Legs up crunches REST :30	Circuit: 3 x 12 The Swimmer Lying sidebends 6 count crunches V-sits REST :30	Circuit: 3 x 12 Superman Reverse crunches Tilt-ups—legs straight Legs up crunches REST :30	Timed curl-ups 1 x :90(:60) 2 x :60 (:60) 1 x :30
Distance run 1.5 mile	Power walk 40:00	Distance run 1.5 mile	

Expert Week 3

TRAINING DAY 1	TRAINING DAY 2	TRAINING DAY 3	TRAINING DAY 4
Circuit: 3x 15 Superman V-sits Hanging leg raises—knees bent Single leg crunches REST :30	Circuit: 3x 15 Flutter kicks Tiltups—legs straight 6 count crunches V-sits REST :30	Circuit: 3x 15 Superman V-sits Hanging leg raises—knees bent Single leg crunches REST :30	Circuit: 3x 15 Flutter kicks Tiltups—legs straight 6 count crunches V-sits REST :30
Interval Sprints 2 x 25 yds @moderate (walk 25 yds) 4 x 50 yds @moderate (walk 25 yds) 2 x 50 yds @fast (walk 25 yds) 1 x 25 yds @moderate (walk 25 yds) 2 x 25 yds @fast (walk 25 yds) 2 x 75 yds @moderate (walk 25 yds)	Distance Run w/hills 1 mile flat 4 x uphill OR stairs (moderate run down) 1 mile flat	Interval Sprints 2 x 25 yds @moderate (walk 25 yds) 4 x 50 yds @moderate (walk 25 yds) 2 x 50 yds @fast (walk 25 yds) 1 x 25 yds @moderate (walk 25 yds) 2 x 25 yds @fast (walk 25 yds) 2 x 75 yds @moderate (walk 25 yds)	

Expert Week 4

TRAINING DAY 1	TRAINING DAY 2	TRAINING DAY 3	TRAINING DAY 4
Circuit: 3x 15 Superman V-sits Hanging leg raises—knees bent Single leg crunches REST :30	Circuit: 3x 15 Flutter kicks Tiltups—legs straight 6 count crunches V-sits REST :30	Circuit: 3x 15 Superman V-sits Hanging leg raises—knees bent Single leg crunches REST :30	**PROGRESS CHECK**
			Ground zero Estimate
Distance Run 2 miles		Distance Run 2 miles	Timed curl-ups 1 x :60
			Interval Sprints 3x 25 yds @moderate (walk 25 yds) 4 x 25 yds@fast (walk 25 yds) 3 x 50 yds @moderate (walk 25 yds) 3 x 50 yds @fast (walk 25 yds) 1 x 100 yds @moderate (walk 25 yds) 1 x 50 yds @fast (walk 25 yds) 1 x 25 yds@fast (walk 25 yds)

Expert Week 5

TRAINING DAY 1	TRAINING DAY 2	TRAINING DAY 3	TRAINING DAY 4
Circuit: 3x 15	Circuit: 3x 15	Circuit: 3x 15	Circuit: 3x 15
Hanging leg raises-knees bent OR Bench V-sits (knees bent)	V-sits—legs straight	Hanging leg raises-knees bent OR Bench V-sits (knees bent)	V-sits—legs straight
6 count crunches	Total body crunches	6 count crunches	Total body crunches
Flutter kicks	4 count crunches	Flutter kicks	4 count crunches
Legs up crunches	Legs up crunches	Legs up crunches	Legs up crunches
REST :30	REST :30	REST :30	REST :30
Distance Run 2.5 miles		Distance Run 2.5 miles	Distance Run w/hills Run 1.5 mile flat 5 x uphill OR stairs (moderate run down) Run 1 mile flat

Expert Week 6

TRAINING DAY 1	TRAINING DAY 2	TRAINING DAY 3	TRAINING DAY 4
Circuit: 4x 15	Circuit: 4x 15	Circuit: 4x 15	Circuit: 4x 15
Hanging leg raises-knees bent OR Bench V-sits (knees bent)	The Swimmer	Hanging leg raises-knees bent OR Bench V-sits (knees bent)	The Swimmer
6 count crunches	Tiltups-knees bent	6 count crunches	Tiltups-knees bent
Flutter kicks	4 count crunches	Flutter kicks	4 count crunches
Legs up crunches	Legs up Crunches	Legs up crunches	Legs up Crunches
REST :30	REST :30	REST :30	REST :30
Power Walk 45:00	Distance Run 3 miles	Power Walk 45:00	Timed curl-ups 1 x 2:00 (:90) 1 x :90 (:90) 1 x :60 (:60) x :30 (:30)

Expert Week 7

TRAINING DAY 1	TRAINING DAY 2	TRAINING DAY 3	TRAINING DAY 4
Circuit: 4x 15 Hanging leg raises (legs straight) OR Bench v-sits (legs straight) Flutter kicks Single leg crunches Side V-bends REST :30	Circuit: 4x 15 Hanging leg raises— side to side OR Bench v-sits- knees bent Tilt-ups—legs straight Total body crunches Legs up crunches REST :30	Circuit: 4x 15 Hanging leg raises (legs straight) OR Bench v-sits (legs straight) Flutter kicks Single leg crunches Side V-bends REST :30	Circuit: 4x 15 Hanging leg raises— side to side OR Bench v-sits- knees bent Tilt-ups—legs straight Total body crunches Legs up crunches REST :30
Distance Run 3 miles	Run w/Hills Run 1.5 mile flat 5 x uphill OR stairs (moderate run down) 1.5 mile flat	Distance Run 3 miles	

Expert Week 8

TRAINING DAY 1	TRAINING DAY 2	TRAINING DAY 3	TRAINING DAY 4
Circuit: 4 x 15 Hanging leg raises (legs straight) OR Bench v-sits (legs straight) Flutter kicks Single leg crunches Side V-bends REST :30	Circuit: 4x 15 Hanging leg raises— side to side OR Bench v-sits- knees bent Tilt-ups—legs straight Total body crunches Legs up crunches REST :30	Circuit: 4 x 15 Hanging leg raises (legs straight) OR Bench v-sits (legs straight) Flutter kicks Single leg crunches Side V-bends REST :30	**PROGRESS CHECK** Ground Zero Estimate
Distance Run w/Intervals 4 x _ mile @moderate + 1/4 mile @fast	Interval Sprints 3x 25 yds @moderate (walk 25 yds) 4x 25 yds@fast (walk 25 yds) 2 x 50 yds @moderate (walk 25 yds) 2 x 50 yds @fast (walk 25 yds) 2 x 75 yds @moderate (walk 25 yds) 1 x 100 yds @fast	Distance Run w/Intervals 4 x _ mile @moderate + 1/4 mile @fast	Timed curl-ups 1 x 2:00

bibliography

Books and Articles

> Baechle, Thomas and Earle. R*oger Essentials of Strength Training and Conditioning.* 2d ed. Champaign, IL: Human Kinetics, 2000.

> Colgan, M. *Optimum Sports Nutrition.* New York: Advanced Research Press, 1993.

> Gray, Henry. *Anatomy of the Human Body.* 20th ed., thoroughly rev. and re-edited by Warren H. Lewis. Philadelphia: Lea & Febiger, 1918. Bartleby.com, 2000, http://www.bartleby.com/107/

> Martini, F., Welch, K. *Fundamentals of Anatomy & Physiology.* 4th ed. Upper Saddle River, NJ: Prentice-Hall, Inc., 1998.

> "The Recommended Quantity and Quality of Exercise for Developing and Maintaining Cardiorespiratory and Muscular Fitness in Healthy Adults." American College of Sports Medicine. Indianapolis: Position Stand, 1990.

> Williams, Melvin H. *Nutrition for Health, Fitness, and Sport.* 5th ed. New York: McGraw-Hill, 1998.

Web Resources

> National Institutes of Health, Washington, D.C. http://www.nih/gov

> National Weight Control Registry. Lifespan, Providence, RI. http://www.lifespan.org/services/bmed/wt_loss/nwcr/

> Strength Training Guidelines. Georgia State University, Department of Kinesiology and Health, Atlanta. http://www.gsu.edu/~wwwfit/strength.html

> Various scientific journal articles. Medline, a division of WebMD, NY. http://www.medscape.com

author bio

Charla is a Certified Strength and Conditioning Specialist with twenty years of strength training and personal training experience. For the past eight years, she has operated FitBoot—Basic Training for Professionals, helping elite athletes and novices achieve balanced conditioning and superior performance using military techniques, which Charla learned as a U.S. Marine Corps officer, and currently accepted athletic conditioning guidelines. The program has received accolades from clients and the media in the Greater Boston area for its "no frills approach" to encouraging every athlete to "give more of themselves physically and emotionally than they ever thought possible."

Training emphasis: Complete conditioning—strength, agility, flexibility, endurance

Areas of experience:

> **Strength training with and without apparatus**

> **Basic nutrition counselling**

> **Athletic/performance conditioning, specifically for general health, martial arts, military and law enforcement, and recreational multi-sport athletes**

> **Special populations—children (from preschool to late adolescents)**

Personal passions: weight training for physique development

Training motto: *mens sana in corpore sano* (a sound mind in a sound body)

She has bee featured on *Chronicle* and *Fox News*, on several radio shows, and in the *Boston Herald*.

also from fair winds

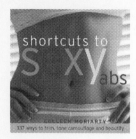

SHORTCUTS TO SEXY ABS
By Colleen Moriarty
ISBN: 1-59233-069-X
$9.95/$13.95 CAN
Paperback; 256 pages
Available wherever books are sold

SEXY ABS THE EASY WAY

With low-rise jeans, belly rings, and bikinis back in style, you need abs like a dancer—curvy on the sides and flat in front.

It's not as hard as you might think! With the 337 belly-busting tips, tricks, and techniques in this engaging how-to book, you will trim your torso faster than you can say *no more baby fat*.

No matter what your age or fitness level, you can beat the big belly blues just in time for that big date, job interview, or trip to the Bahamas. From Pilates to no-bloat eating plans, you'll find all the fitness, beauty, fashion, and diet shortcuts you need, including:

- The Great Date Plan
- The Look Marvelous at the Office Plan
- The Fabulous Party Plan
- The Get Your Abs Back After Pregnancy Plan
- The Bikini Beach Plan

Everything you need to know about great-looking abs is here. With *Shortcuts to Sexy Abs* as your guide, you'll give every belly dancer and ballerina a run for her money.

also from fair winds

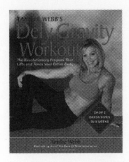

TAMILEE WEBB'S DEFY GRAVITY WORKOUT
By Tamilee Webb
ISBN: 1-59233-087-8
$19.95/£12.99/$28.95
Paperback; 192 pages
Available wherever books are sold

FIGHT THE SIGNS OF AGING WITH THIS EASY-TO-DO, ONE-OF-A-KIND WORKOUT PROGRAM

Tamilee Webb, star of the best-selling *Buns of Steel* video series has created a plan designed to fight sagging and age-related weight gain. This fat-burning, body-lifting program features walking and resistance exercises that will give you a younger-looking body in just eight weeks.

By following this program, you will:
- burn fat
- lift your butt, trim your thighs, and flatten your belly
- develop a leaner, longer body than you've seen in years
- drop two dress sizes in eight weeks

Like her devoted fans, Tamilee Webb needed to change her workout routine as she got older in order to continue seeing results and fight the natural pull of gravity. She created the workout routines in this book to focus on lifting and sculpting a firmer, more youthful body.

also from fair winds

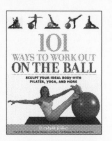

101 WAYS TO WORK OUT ON THE BALL
By Elizabeth Gillies
ISBN: 1-59233-084-3
$19.95/£12.99/$28.95
Paperback; 176 pages
Available wherever books are sold

SCULPT YOUR IDEAL BODY WITH PILATES, YOGA, AND MORE

Everyone loves the workout ball! It can help with weight training, Pilates, yoga, and even cardio and stretching moves. And nobody knows the ball like Liz Gillies. *101 Ways to Work Out on the Ball* gives you exercises that will strengthen, lengthen, tone, and stretch your body like no other form of exercise can. The moves will work for beginners, intermediate, and advanced exercisers; some even require weights to sculpt your arms and legs while strengthening your core. The program includes workout plans and tips for progressing through the series.

Liz Gillies stars in numerous videos including *Zone Pilates, Stability Ball Workouts, Stability Ball for Dummies*, and most recently her own "Core Fitness" line of videos. She is the owner and artistic director of The Insidescoop Studio in New York, where she has been certifying teachers in the Pilates Method since 1997. She is regularly featured in news programs and national publications.

also from fair winds

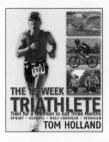

THE 12-WEEK TRIATHLETE
By Tom Holland
ISBN: 1-59233-126-2
$17.95/£11.99/$24.95
Paperback; 256 pages
Available wherever books are sold

IT ONLY TAKES 12 WEEKS TO TRAIN TO COMPETE IN A
TRIATHLON—NO MATTER WHAT LEVEL YOU'RE AT NOW

Tom Holland, who has competed in ten Ironman races, fourteen
marathons, and trained hundreds of athletes around the world, will
give you all the information and techniques you need to feel confi-
dent and enjoy your next race. The training programs will help you
reach your goals, whether it's your first competition or you're a vet-
eran racer looking to improve your time and the quality of your
skills.

You'll get helpful, sport-specific insight on every type of triathlon,
including Sprint, Olympic, Half-Ironman, and Ironman.

Tom Holland is an accomplished triathlete and a member of
PowerBar Team Elite. A certified trainer and presenter, he is the
author of *The Truth About How to Get in Shape* and creator of three
exercise videos, including *Tom Holland's Total Body Workout II*,
Tom Holland's Total Ab Workouts, and *Tom Holland's Total Body
Workout*.

MAKE SURE YOU STAY IN STEP!

You have the game plan
Now get the coaching that keeps you...
Focused. Motivated. Improving.

ACHIEVING!

GREATER BOSTON

One-to-One Training

At your location
Home. Office. Park. Gym. *

* Where permitted

WORLD WIDE

FitbyFone

Long distance coaching
Nutrition Guidance.
Customized Program.

BOSTON

**FitBoot – Basic Training
for Professionals**

New England's original boot
camp fitness program
Structure. Discipline.
Accountability.

RESULTS

CONTACT US TODAY

1-877-FITBOOT   www.fitboot.com